MW01232505

INTERMITTENT FASTING

for Women

A SIMPLE GUIDE TO GET STARTED AND ACHIEVE
QUICK RESULTS AND BENEFITS.
LOSE WEIGHT, BURN FAT, AND IMPROVE
QUALITY OF LIFE THROUGH THE PROCESS OF
METABOLIC AUTOPHAGY

KELLY ALLEN

4

Table of Contents

Introduction

In this book, we will be talking about how to follow intermittent fasting and how you can benefit from it. Most of the time, people start following intermittent fasting only because they are looking to change the way their body functions or to achieve a particular look but the truth is intermittent fasting is way more than that.

As you read along, you will see how important it is to follow intermittent fasting, and how it can help you to achieve your goal, whether it is to lose weight or gain muscle. Even though intermittent fasting is very straightforward for men, it is crucial that you take care of some side effects you might face if you are women. Make sure that you understand how intermittent fasting works for women, and how to execute it the right way. Which is what we will be helping you with specifically when it comes to following intermittent fasting and what it can do for you.

As you read along, we will talk about things which you have never heard of when it comes to intermittent fasting and women, and we will also talk about how to follow intermittent fasting if you are women. Since most of the time, people don't talk about this, and it is imperative that we do. With that being said, I hope you enjoy this book and learn a lot from it as we put the effort in to produce the best content possible.

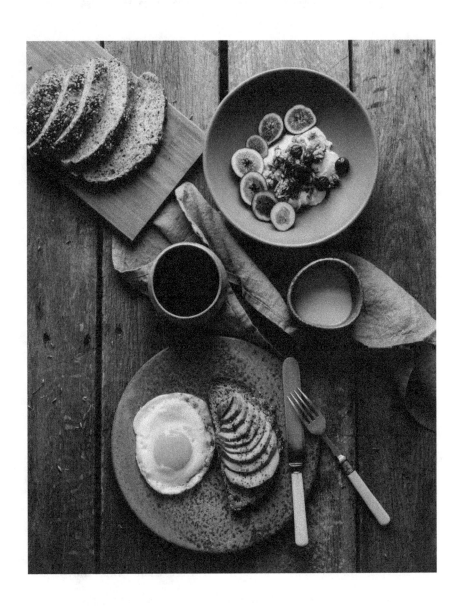

Chapter 1: What is Intermittent Fasting

For people wondering what intermittent fasting is, it is essentially an eating protocol where you will be fasting or not eating for hours at a time, to even day. Think of intermittent fasting as a cyclical way of consuming calories instead of eating a specific type of food and to see benefits from the meal. Nonetheless, intermittent fasting has been known to be one of the top eating protocols for some time now. Later on, in this book, we will further discuss the benefits of intermittent fasting and the different methods you can follow to achieve your goal of health and wellness. However, before we do that let's talk about intermittent fasting a bit and its history

Intermittent fasting has been in practice for a long time now. Although many fitness experts have recently popularized it, it has been followed by humanity for thousands of years now. As we talked about this before, many religions have been following fasting for the ritual ceremonies. Earlier age ancestors also followed fasting, not intentionally but none the less they did.

Which makes me wonder, why were ancestors healthier than us. Even though their life expectancy was a lot shorter than ours, they still managed to avoid diseases like obesity and diabetes. Some might say that fasting had a considerable role to play on that, so in this chapter, we will talk about the backstory of how intermittent fasting started. It is imperative to know about the backstory, as it makes you understand better. Without further Ado, let's talk about it.

The back story of intermittent fasting

Fasting can be traced back thousands of years back and was used to treat illness and fix diseases. Fasting was considered a healing tradition in the earlier days, and Hippocrates also used it. One of the treatments he prescribed was too fast, and he also wrote: "to eat when you are sick, is to feed the illness."

Moreover, the ancient Greek writer Plutarch also wrote: "instead of using medicine, better fast today." Most of the ancient Greek thinkers were a firm believer in fasting for better health. Many Biblical scholars believed in fixing diseases/illness internally, and fasting was one of the essential medicines prescribed by them. Their theory goes as once you get sick, you have no desire to eat, which is a sign from your body, to hold off on the eating part. Ancient Greeks also believed that it improved brain function, which is true.

Think about it, when was the last time you had burger and pizza and noticing mental fog and lethargy right after. It is prevalent to see these symptoms when you overeat, and when you overeat, your blood is transferred to your intestine from your brain to cope with the food, which is the main reason why people notice the mental fog after eating high-calorie foods. Besides the Greeks there where many other firm believers of fasting. The founding fathers of the United States of

America, Benjamin Franklin once said: "The best of all medicine is resting and fasting."

As you know, many religions, such as Muslim, Christian, and Buddha, believed in the healing powers of fasting. They used it to cleanse and purify the soul, which makes sense since fasting has shown to detoxify the body. Fast forward to 2006, when Martin Berkhan created intermittent fasting. The reason why he created it was simple; it was to save time and money cooking. This decision of his, made him lose body fat balance out hormone and live an overall healthy lifestyle.

The method he used was the 16/8 method, which is the most popular method for intermittent fasting. Later down the road in 2012, intermittent fasting started to get some further notice. Harvard University, which is one of the most renown university out there wrote an article on intermittent fasting. It stated all the intermittent fasting benefit brings with it, such as weight loss and hormone balance.

Numerous fitness professionals have now popularized intermittent fasting, and they say it is the best way to eat throughout the day. However, they don't realize that intermittent fasting has been here for a long time now. Many successful people live by intermittent fasting, and the reason is simple. When you start intermittent fasting, you will think and perform better. According to ancient Greek thinkers, it will help you heal from illness as well. So now you know the history of intermittent fasting.

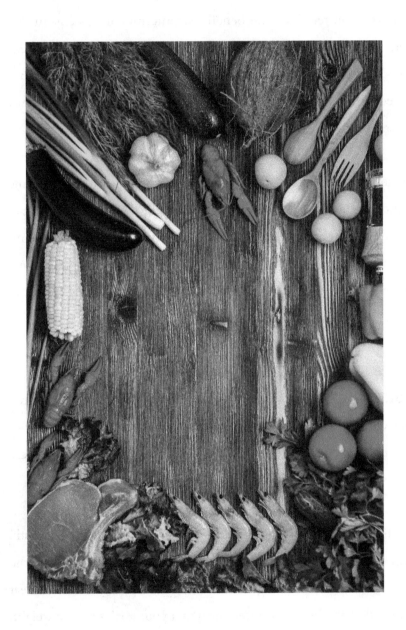

Why is intermittent fasting superior:

Many people know that intermittent fasting is superior to most diets out there, as you can tell from the benefits of intermittent fasting. In this chapter, we will go into more depths on how superior intermittent fasting is, and it is not just healthy for you physically but in many other ways. People who follow regular diets don't realize how much money they spend on food.

Let's take the paleo diet; for example, you're supposed to buy organic fruits and vegetables and organic meat on top of that. Which could get very expensive, as compared to intermittent fasting where there are no restrictions on what kind of food you will be eating it is only time-based. Let me speak from personal example, I use to follow the Paleo Diet, and I would spend around $300 a week on groceries.

Ever since I started following intermittent fasting, my spending went down $150 a week, which is a lot of money saved and could be invested in other ventures. If you're looking to save money then highly consider intermittent fasting, another benefit of intermittent fasting is that there are no restrictions on what kind of food you can eat.

Although I don't recommend you eat pizzas and burgers, you can still get away with eating most of the foods you want while still enjoying the benefits of intermittent fasting. I would always recommend that you eat in a caloric deficit while intermittent fasting if your goal is to lose weight, the wonderful thing about intermittent fasting is that it will be easy for you to eat in a caloric deficit since you only have a little time to eat. Another thing that makes intermittent fasting more superior than other diets is the time you save not eating. Most of you don't realize how much time we spend eating when your intermittent fasting you will recognize much more time you have to do more work or other activities you want to take part in. Meaning if you're working and you want to get the job done quicker, you will be able to as you 'don't have to worry about eating just yet.

If you have a busy work life, then intermittent fasting might be the answer for you as it will be saving a lot of time getting work rather than following your diet. What we just touched upon, were merely the lifestyle benefits you will get from intermittent fasting. Having lifestyle benefits with a diet is a great thing to have, and that is one of the reasons why intermittent fasting is more superior than other diets. Moving on, we will talk about how intermittent fasting is superior to different diets in regards to health and wellness.

As you know, already intermittent fasting helps you balance out your hormones, and it also helps you with detoxifying your body. Since most diets make you feel underfed and sluggish throughout the day, with intermittent fasting, it was the complete opposite. When you're following intermittent fasting, you will start to notice that your brain function has been enhanced, you will see that your focus and mental energy has gone up. The reason behind it is that your insulin doesn't spike up randomly throughout the day as it would when you're following a regular diet, which causes you to stay more focused at work or anything else that you are doing.

The most significant benefit of intermittent fasting I noticed was that I didn't have to meal prep every day. I hate meal prepping, and intermittent fasting gave me the freedom to not do so. I would just fast throughout the day, and when I would come back home, I would break my fast. This was the best thing ever, and intermittent fasting gives you a lot of time at your hand to do the more essential things.

Which was a significant plus for intermittent fasting and made it a lot more superior than other diets for me and hopefully for you as well. All the health benefits you get from fasting, such as the lowered risk of heart disease and diabetes has been proven scientifically as compared to most other diets which haven't been tested with proper science, which makes intermittent fasting a lot more Superior than different foods in all aspects.

Now, if you want to know why intermittent fasting is a lot more Superior than other diets, then let's recap. Intermittent fasting saves money, it helps you think better, it gives you more time, more freedom to eat whatever you want, and it gives you all the health benefits prevention from diseases. All these benefits I just listed is the reason why you are trying to live a healthier life. You want the free time, you want the mental clarity, and you want the prevention from illness and diseases.

If you want it all, then intermittent fasting is your answer. That is the reason why intermittent fasting more superior than other diets out there. Intermittent fasting provides you with a bunch of positives when compared to different diets, and I highly doubt that there is any other diet out there which will help you save time and money most of the time it is the complete opposite. Everything from health benefits, hormone balance, and lifestyle benefits make intermittent fasting an absolute winner, also making it more superior than other diets out there.

The science behind intermittent fasting:

In the beginning, intermittent fasting was created to lose body fat and look better aesthetically. Nonetheless, there is some science behind the theory of intermittent fasting, which we will be covering in the section of the book the science behind intermittent fasting. The most common argument used to justify the science behind intermittent fasting is from the evolutionary standpoint. As we talked about it before, our ancestors used to fast unintentionally.

They did that because they wouldn't have access to food as we do in the modern day. It's said that we digest and utilize foods better when we are in a fasting state, as it is what we used to do in the earlier days. Because of our ancestors, we tend to metabolize food much better after a prolonged period of fasting. This theory is the most popular theory based on intermittent fasting, and that is what most fitness professionals talk about in terms of why fasting works great on people.

Although there is some truth to this theory, there is still some science to be talked about. By now, you should be aware of the hormone benefits you get from intermittent fasting, especially with insulin. Now to break down the effects of insulin with fasting, here is how it works. When your fasting throughout the day, your insulin will stay flat, meaning it won't spike up or down.

What this will do is help you use fat for energy instead of glycogen, most of the time, people burn glycogen first, which tends to be the food they had just eaten before they burn fat. What intermittent fasting allows you to do is use fat straight away for energy instead of using glycogen, making it very good for fat loss. Even though fasting has almost the same effects on women and men, there's still some difference. Women will notice more hunger than men when they're fasting; the reason why women will notice more hunger as compared men is because of their reproductive system.

Compared to men, 'women's body tends to hold more stored energy, and it is merely because they have to carry a baby. Which would make fasting a bit more tough for women than men if done for a prolonged period of time, this is more of a heads up than anything. For women, we recommend starting with a shorter fast and eventually build up to a longer one. There are a lot of benefits to fasting for a prolonged period of time, after 16 hours of fasting cell rejuvenation takes place. When you are fasting, there is something in your body, which occurs known as autophagy. It is a process when your body destroys your old cells and rejuvenates itself with new cells, and this process makes your body produce stronger and efficient cells.

Which gives you hosts of benefits such as better skin, better heart health, and anti-aging properties. This makes it an excellent choice for someone who's also looking for better health and well-being. We will talk about autophagy in more length later in this book. We previously talked about insulin and how it stays flat throughout the day when you're fasting; this makes it a great way to boost your growth hormone while you're fasting.

You see, insulin and growth hormone don't go hand-in-hand if your growth hormone spiking up chances are insulin's down, and if your insulin spiking up the probability to your growth hormone is down.

When your fasting your growth hormone can increase up to 4000%, giving you a host of benefits, as you know, growth hormone helps you burn fat and also helps with anti-aging. Having a higher amount of growth hormone in your body is a must if you're looking to burn fat and to feel better throughout the day. One of the better benefits of intermittent fasting is the mental focus you get from it. When your fasting, you are going to survival mode, which makes you go on a fight or flight instinct.

This instinct you notice a boost in, helps you focus a lot better at the task at hand, making you more productive when you're in a fasting state. Which means, if your goal is to get more stuff done and to be more productive throughout the day, then there's no better way to go about it than fasting. The science behind intermittent fasting is this, from a fat loss standpoint, you will be burning a lot more fat than glycogen. As you know, when you're following a regular diet and regular eating throughout the day, your glycogen stores are higher, which means your body will attack the glycogen before it attacks the fat. What intermittent fasting does, is an attack or burn the fat from the get-go, making it optimal for fat loss.

From a hormone standpoint, your insulin will be more flatlined. Making you less prone to type 2 diabetes overall help you burn more fat, and you will also notice your growth hormone go up, which will lead to anti-aging properties. Another thing which we talked about is cell rejuvenation, which makes your body get rid of the bad cells and rejuvenate with better and stronger cells.

Finally, fasting gets you into starvation mode, which activates your fight or flight instinct. This instinct helps you to focus more, and to get things done whether you want to do or have to do. By now, you know the science behind intermittent fasting, and why it is better suited for most people. We will talk about more of the benefits of intermittent fasting later in the book. But for now, we just wanted to cover the science behind it.

By now, you have learned most of the basics of intermittent fasting, you have learned how fasting works in your body. You also know how fasting helps you with better health and overall well-being, and now we will get into the different types of fasting methods and their specific benefits. Every fasting process is executed for a reason, and there is a different way to fast if your goal is to feel healthier and more productive. There is a modified fast for all needs, even though they all provide health and weight-loss benefits. Some fasts are more suited for fat loss, and others are more suited for cell rejuvenation. More on that in the next chapter, until then.

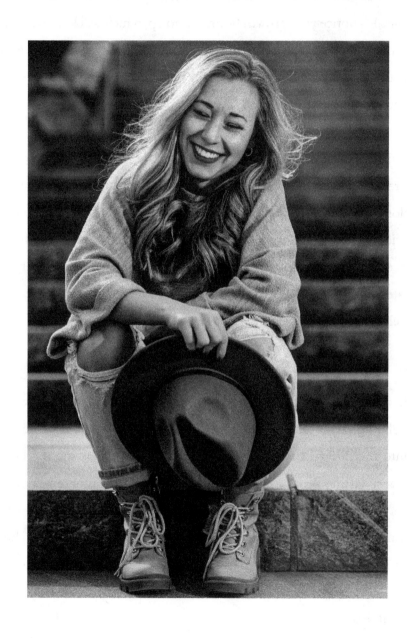

Chapter 2: Benefits of Intermittent Fasting

We have talked about many concerns and side effects related to intermittent fasting in detail, but now let's talk about the health benefits in further length. Many people know there are numerous benefits to intermittent fasting; the major ones are weight loss and cell rejuvenation. Even though these are great benefits, there are many more which intermittent fasting provides you with.

In this chapter, we will go over benefits that come along intermittent fasting. There are many compelling benefits which you might not even know about, so we will go step by step thru each interest. If you are iffy about starting intermittent fasting, then this chapter might turn you on to the idea of fasting. Without wasting any more time, let's talk about the positives of intermittent fasting and how it can help you.

Weight-loss in a healthy manner

As you know, there are many ways to lose weight. However, one of the most popular methods being used to lose weight is intermittent fasting, and there is a good reason behind it. Many people don't know this, but intermittent fasting is perhaps the best way for someone to lose "body fat" instead of "body-weight." When following most diets, followers tend to lose a ton of weight, but most of the time it is muscle and water weight they are losing.

On the other hand, intermittent fasting makes you lose more body fat. Here is how it works, when you are fasting for a prolonged period of time you have burned out all your glycogen stores. Which makes the body hit your reserves, and that of course, is your body fat. You will be burning more body fat, instead of muscle mass or glycogen, which makes it ideal for people looking to lose weight. Also, as you know, intermittent fasting plays a huge role in affecting your hormones. Your insulin will flatline, and your growth hormone will go up, this will prime your body to burn body fat instead and will do so in a healthy manner.

Now the main reason why intermittent fasting works is pretty simple when you break your fast you have a tiny eating window. This allows you to stay in a caloric deficit, which makes you lose weight in the long run. Unless you binge eat, you will healthily lose weight. According to a 2014 study, people following intermittent fasting lost a significant amount of body weight. Intermittent fasting was found to reduce weight by 3-8% over the period of 3-24 weeks. When examined even further, the participants lost 0.55 lbs. a week on average. However, participants who followed the alternative day fasting lost 1.65 pounds a week, making it a much better-suited tool for people looking to lose weight.

Another way intermittent fasting is healthier when compared to other weight loss diets is the fact that there are no restrictions on foods. When people follow different diets, it makes it very hard for them to follow since they have to eat every two hours and many other jargons, intermittent fasting makes it very simple for you as there isn't a lot to think about. Where different diets make your weight loss goals your job, intermittent fasting makes it super easy for you, and this makes intermittent fasting a healthy and sustainable way to lose body weight. Overall, intermittent fasting is a very healthy and sustainable way to lose body-fat. If you are looking to get rid of excess body fat, then you have nothing else to look for, intermittent fasting is the answer for you. Besides weight loss, intermittent fasting comes with other benefits, which we already talked about. However, now we will go into further details of the health benefits intermittent fasting comes with when you start.

Increased longevity

There have been many studies showing that intermittent fasting can boost longevity. As you might know by now that fasting can help with cell rejuvenation or also known as autophagy, this process enables you to get rid of the old and weak cell and replace it with newer stronger ones. This process has shown to increase longevity and overall well-being, which is one of the reasons why intermittent fasting can help you live a longer life. Moreover, some studies are showing that reducing calories in animals by 30% to 40% has shown to increase their lifespan. However, there is no study done on humans claiming such. Nonetheless, some studies are suggesting that monkeys that ate less lived longer. However, there was another study indicating that it wasn't the case on a 25-year-old long study done by another party.

Although there is no actual study backing these claims up, it does show that people who ate less had a fewer risk of diseases which could lead to longevity. Which is excellent news when looking at it from that angle, there is a lot of disease prevention that comes with intermittent fasting, but we will talk about those later in this chapter. However, the main thing to remember would be the fact that intermittent fasting helps with autophagy, which enables you to rejuvenate cells. This makes it very evident that intermittent fasting can help you with longevity and overall well-being, which is a great thing to consider.

Prevent diseases

There are many diseases present in today's day and age, and it very common to meet someone suffering from one. Which means, we need to figure out a way to reduce the risk of diseases for overall health and well-being. Intermittent has shown to lower risk of many diseases, and we will be discussing all the diseases intermittent fasting can help get rid. Two of the many diseases intermittent fasting could help manage are Alzheimer's and Parkinson's.

As you know, intermittent fasting helps to boost brain health and to lower the risk of neurogenic diseases. Some studies are showing that intermittent fasting can help reduce the risk of depression, even though some people might not consider this a condition, it is still a significant issue in our society. Intermittent fasting has also shown to reduce cholesterol, a 2010 study on overweight women found that fasting improved hosts of health complications including cholesterol levels (LDL) and blood pressure which is also known as the silent killer.

Intermittent fasting also helps with reducing type 2 diabetes, and there was one study done on men, which showed that intermittent fasting helped them stop insulin treatment. Although we don't recommend, you try this if you have type 2 diabetes, that goes to show you the power of intermittent fasting and insulin resistance.

Nonetheless, many studies are suggesting that intermittent fasting can lower the risk of diabetes. Another devastating disease which intermittent fasting helps getting rid of would be heart diseases. As you know, intermittent fasting enables you to get rid of hypertension, which leads to heart issues. Once your blood pressure goes down, your heart will be working a lot more efficiently, allowing you a healthier life.

In regards to a healthier life, intermittent fasting has also shown to reduce the risk of obesity. One study done on obese women suggested that intermittent fasting reduced the risk of obesity in women, which makes sense as it helps you lose and manage body weight. One of the main diseases which intermittent fasting could help reduce the risk of is cancer, even though it hasn't been proven yet. Many scientists believe fasting for a prolonged period could help you get rid of cancer.

These facts about intermittent fasting show you how intermittent fasting can help you get free of many diseases, and some have been backed up with concrete studies, whereas others are still being researched.

Nonetheless, you can't say that about other diets out there. Intermittent fasting will help you to get rid of many things and prevent you from further having any diseases. There is no better way of getting rid of illness or problems without the use of modern medicine, and intermittent fasting is so powerful that it will also boost your immune system which will help you avoid small issues like the common flu. All in all, there are many rejuvenating properties which come along with intermittent fasting, so don't overlook it and keep all the positives in mind before you look at the negatives.

Reduce stress and inflammation

Intermittent fasting has shown a significant reduction in inflammation. As you know, information causes a lot of many chronic diseases such as Alzheimer's, dementia, obesity, diabetes, and much more. Now, there are many ways that intermittent fasting helps you get rid of inflammation. The first one being autophagy, as you know intermittent fasting helps you with cell rejuvenation cleans up itself by eating out the old self and rejuvenating them with the newer stronger ones. If your body does not rejuvenate itself with more modern cells, the older ones have stayed for an extended period of time can cause inflammation.

As you know, the average diet does not allow for cell rejuvenation to happen; this is where intermittent fasting comes in as it has been proven to help with the process of autophagy. Another way intermittent fasting enables you to get rid of inflammation would be by producing ketones. When you are fasting, your body uses up all the glycogen stores, which makes it start using stored fat for fuel, and when fats are broken down for energy ketones are produced. One of the most popular ketones in your body will block a part of your immune system, which is responsible for inflammatory disorders. Another way intermittent fasting helps you lower the risk of inflammation is by making you insulin sensitive, and when your body becomes insulin resistant, you will be holding much glucose in your bloodstream. More glucose in your blood will create inflammation, and intermittent fasting allows your body to get rid of all the glucose, which helps you reduce inflammation in your body.

Now that we've talked about many ways intermittent fasting enables you to reduce inflammation, let's talk about how intermittent fasting can help you get rid of stress. You see, inflammation and stress go hand in hand. If you have high levels of inflammation, chances are your stress levels are going to be higher. Which means that if you lower your inflammation, you will reduce your stress levels, and as you know, fasting helps with better brain function. Intermittent fasting enables you to send better signals to your brain, which would equal a better functioning brain.

When your mind is functioning at its utmost peak, your levels of stress drop down. Better brain function will also help you get rid of any stress you might be having, and having overall better health can help you reduce stress. Overall, all the health benefits you get from intermittent fasting will help you get rid of your stress or at least lower it. Which means, even if you are not facing stress, intermittent fasting will help you have a better functioning brain and also help you get rid of any mental fog or stress you might be dealing. What that in mind, always make sure you consult a physician if you are noticing much more stress than you can handle, as it can be something severe and not fixable by intermittent fasting.

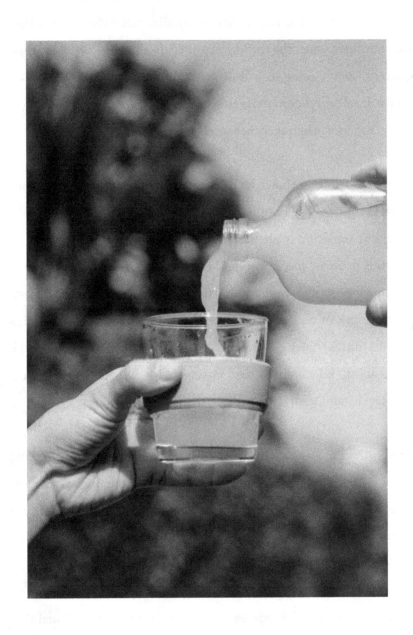

Body detox and cell cleaned

Detoxing your body is very important when it comes to living a long healthy life, many people detox their body thru juice cleanse or other methods out there when the truth is that they don't work. Time and time again, intermittent fasting has shown to help detox your body in both the cellular level and digestive level, which means intermittent fasting is a lot more superior when it comes to cleaning your body.

As you know, from a cellular level intermittent fasting detoxifies your body with the process of autophagy, what this process does it eat out the bad cells and replace it with healthier and much more stronger cells. Through this process, you will notice benefits such as a stronger immune system, prevention of diseases, and insulin sensitivity. It has also shown to reduce the risk of cancer, which is a great thing to know. Overall, this is how intermittent fasting detoxifies your body from a cellular level. Let's talk about how intermittent fasting helps you detoxify from a digestive level standpoint.

People say that your gut is your second brain, and studies are showing how your stomach and mind are connected. Which means if your digestive system isn't functioning at its utmost peak, then chances are your brain won't either. It is very important to have a gut which is clean and working correctly, and intermittent helps a lot with this process.

It has been shown that intermittent fasting can help you clean out your gut and intestines out of debris and junk. Sometimes, it is essential that we give your digestive system a break from eating all those foods regularly. Once you start your fast your body will begin to slowly get rid of all the toxins present in your gut, you see when you are eating all the time your body doesn't get a chance to clean itself.

Your body has to focus on digesting the food instead of cleaning out the toxins when you give your body a break from eating; it will start to clean out its gut. Which makes this process great for people who are fasting, when you have a high functioning gut, it will help you digest your food a lot better and also think better. The detoxifying body helps you tremendously with lowering the risk of diseases, which will help you live a longer life.

By now, you can see the pattern; intermittent fasting helps you from every single place to prevent diseases and many other complications. Which means there are more positives than negatives with intermittent fasting, as we go along in this chapter, you will learn more benefits when it comes to intermittent fasting. However, remember that these will only work unless you do, you have to follow intermittent fasting the right way to see these benefits. With that being said, I hope you have learned a lot from this book as we are almost half way through it! Now let's move on to another benefit.

Improved insulin sensitivity

As you know, intermittent fasting helps you get more insulin sensitive, which helps you with many things. To understand it better, let me explain to you how insulin works. Every time you eat a meal, your insulin spikes up, then insulin is used to shuttle food either to muscle or your fat store.

When you have too much glycogen in your bloodstream, your body will send that energy to your fat stores. Whereas if you're insulin sensitive, your body will send the glycogen to muscle stores and will be used for energy. When you are insulin sensitive, you are more likely to use up all the glycogen from your food faster, and not requiring your glycogen to be converted into fats.

How intermittent fasting helps with curing insulin resistance is by using up all the glycogen stores, making your body use up fat stores and when you eat food again, it will use up all the glycogen and shuttle it straight to the muscle mass to be used for energy instead of being stored into fat. That is how intermittent fasting helps you become more insulin sensitive; the benefits of being insulin sensitive are many. Once you become insulin sensitive, you will notice more mental energy and less mental fog, and you will also see less fat being stored in your body which makes it ideal for people looking to lose fat and or gain muscle.

Being insulin sensitive will also help you gain more muscle since most of the energy will be sent out to your muscle stores; it will be used to build stronger muscles instead of storing it into fat. Being insulin sensitive is a must, as it will also help you get rid of possible diseases such as type 2 diabetes. All in all, intermittent fasting helps you tremendously with insulin sensitively, which will overall help you live a healthier life.

Increased production of neurotrophic growth factor

Believe it or not, intermittent fasting affects your brain in a significant way. It all happens from the help of brain-derived neurotrophic growth factor, also known as (BDNF), this helps promote neuroplasticity. Neuroplasticity is your brain's ability to migrate and shapeshift, and this helps our brain to produce new brain cells. Once you have an ample supply of BDNF, we can preserve older cells while producing new brain cells. Which means your brain will be healthy and will keep growing because of the new cells coming. Multiple studies are showing that intermittent fasting to improve brain-derived neurotrophic growth factor, more specifically when it has to do with synapses, this is where your neurotransmitter travel cell to cell.

Fasting has shown to promote this, and there was a study done where it showed fasting for 12 to 16 hours has shown to increase levels of brain-derived neurotrophic growth factor by around 50-400%. Now we know that fasting helps promote (BDNF), more explicitly fasting helps when it comes down to synapses. It improves what is known as synaptic plasticity, and this helps modulate our moods better. For instance, we can strengthen a synapse or weaken a synapse. This process enables you to be in the moment when you need to be happy or scared; this will help you modulate that accordingly.

In layman's term, this process helps us change our mood and be reactive at the moment. For example, if you need to be more focused, you will be able to because you are modulating it. When your brain-derived neurotrophic growth factor increases, so do your (BDNF) expression. This process helps you produce more brain cells and protect more brain cells, and this affects your cells at a genetic level altering our DNA. Which makes fasting one of the best ways to protect your brain, and this gives your brain all the help it needs to preserve and recycle out old cells.

Another thing which it helps with is producing more growth hormone, and there was a study done where it showed upwards of a 4000% increase in growth hormone levels. Which is huge when it comes to improvements, as you know, growth hormone is responsible for many things of them being weight loss. It is a plus to have higher amounts of growth hormone, in both men and women. I know that the information was very scientific, so to put in very simple terms, your brain will rejuvenate a lot quicker.

It will also help you with controlling your moods, which will make it easy to adapt at the moment. Brain-derived neurotrophic growth factor will also help you produce higher levels of growth hormone and serotonin, which are both crucial for mental well-being. Overall, this makes intermittent fasting one of the best brain-improving eating patterns out there. For readers looking for mental clarity and fewer moods swings throughout the day, intermittent fasting is your answer to all.

Boost immune system

There is a reason why having a healthy immune system is very important, as it will help you get less sick and be more "immune" to disease. Intermittent fasting has shown to increase the immune system, so we will talk about how it boosts the immune system. There was a study done on stem cells when it comes down to a fasting individual; more specifically, they took a look at how the stem cells rejuvenated.

The study concluded that intermittent fasting depleted white blood cells, which is precisely what we want so our body can produce better and more efficient cells, which lead to more production of stem cells and lesser of white cells. Once you start to get rid of your old white blood cells, you will start producing new ones, which will overall help you recover faster. This study also found that there was a reduced amount of protein kinase A (PKA), which allows the stem cells to regenerate. If you have a lower amount of (PKA), this means that it will enable the cells to turn on the regeneration mode, which will allow them to create new cells.

As you know, intermittent fasting has shown to reduce insulin levels, which is a great thing for someone looking to boost their immune system. There was a study done showing that high amounts of insulin levels, prevented t cells from doing its job effectively. The t cells are here to suppress inflammation and to fight off illness, t cells are most of the time responsible for getting rid of toxins which cause illness and inflammation. When your insulin levels are high, t cells are not performing at their highest potential, which causes our immune system to drop down.

When you are fasting, there isn't a requirement for insulin spikes, which lets our body help the t cells work at a higher level and overall boosting our immune system. Since you aren't eating for a long time, this will give your gut a break. When you eat a big meal, around 70% of the blood and energy goes to your stomach to digest it. Which means, when you are fasting, you give your body a chance to recover. Everything is healing when you are fasting, which includes the digestive system. Meaning, your gut will be working a lot more effectively once you have given it some time to heal.

As you know, digestion plays a massive role in both our mental health and immune system, about 60% of our immune system is in our colon, which means when you are fasting, you are recovering your whole body and overall boosting your immune system. You will be doing yourself a tremendous service if you can manage to boost your immune system, and with all the backed-up science showing how intermittent fasting can help you promote your immune system and reduce many other health problems, there is no reason not to start intermittent fasting as soon as possible.

More energy and muscle mass increased

Even if your goal isn't to put on more muscle, it is still good to have more muscle mass as it helps you with many things. However, the main thing having higher amounts of muscle mass helps you with would be fat loss; having a higher muscle mass will help you burn more fat since it increases your metabolic rate. Don't worry, and you don't have to look like a bodybuilder for that to happen; nonetheless, it is essential to have the right amount of muscle mass, especially for women.

Intermittent fasting has shown to increase and preserve muscle mass, so let's talk about how that happens. There was a study done between two groups of me one followed a 16/8 fasting method, and the other followed, whereas the other followed a normal eating pattern. Both groups followed the same workout and the same diet, and just the group fasting would eat in the eight-hour window. What they noticed after eight weeks was, both the groups gained and preserved the same amount of muscle, but the group who were following the intermittent fasting lost more fat.

This shows that intermittent fasting not only helped followers gain muscle and preserve it, but it also helped them lose fat simultaneously. The main reason behind that is growth hormone, as you know, intermittent fasting has shown to increase growth hormone in our bodies. What growth hormone mainly does, it allows a lot less muscle breakdown and to burn more fat, which is one of the main reasons why intermittent fasting is so beneficial for building and preserving muscle mass.

Another great benefit of intermittent fasting as you know is higher energy levels, and there is a reason behind it. Many people know how it feels to have a sugar crash, you feel tired and lethargic, and the culprit behind it is insulin. When insulin is spiked up, your energy level goes down as this gives your brain a signal to relax. When you are intermittent fasting, there are no insulin spikes throughout the day, which provides you with more energy to stuff.

Another reason why you have more energy when you are fasting is that your body goes into a fight or flight response and since your body is in a normal starvation mode, it feels like for it to get food it needs to hunt. Which is when your body produces more adrenaline throughout the day, which gives you more energy as you go along. Just be aware, at the beginning of your fasting journey, you might feel less energized.

The reason behind it is because your body is still getting used to these changes, but after a week or two, you should start to notice more energy. Use the energy to get more work done at work and gym. In my opinion, this is the most significant benefit which comes along with intermittent fasting. More energy makes you feel a lot better when you are looking towards making it thru those long days.

These are all the main benefits which come along when you start fasting; the benefits truly outweigh all the negatives fasting might come with. These benefits can be life changing to most people, lowering the risk of diseases and increasing longevity; it's an amazing thing to have. Intermittent fasting provides you with that and then some. It is now time for you to pick a fasting plan and start implementing it, which is what we are going to talk about in the next chapter.

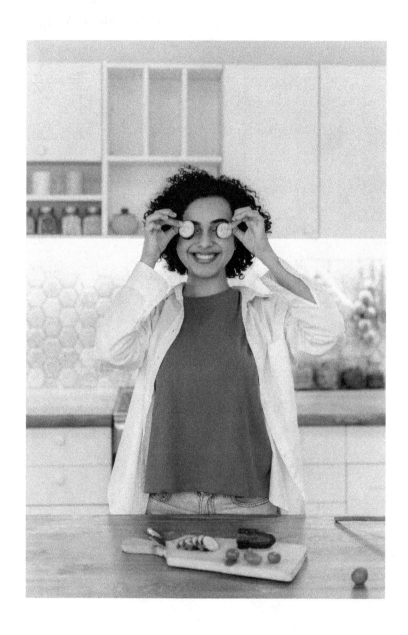

Chapter 3: Different Types of Fasting Methods

Since intermittent fasting has come out, there have been several methods which are being popularized by many fitness experts and gurus. At first, it was the simple fasting strategy which was fast for 16 hours and eat for 8 hours. But since then, we have discovered multiple different ways of fasting which are being used for fat loss and overall well-being.

In today's chapter, we will be talking about the seven main intermittent fasting methods, which are being used by most fitness professional and experts out there. One of the best things in regards to following intermittent fasting is the ability to have choices. When fasting, you have so many ways to go about it that it makes it very user-friendly, as you will learn later on in this chapter. Truthfully if you are deciding to follow intermittent fasting, then you should have no excuse. Intermittent fasting works with you instead of against you, unlike most diets out there.

There are many ways to go about fasting, and we will be talking about those in this chapter. Just remember, even though you might have found the right fasting cycle for your lifestyle needs that doesn't mean it will fit your goal. For instance, if your goal is to notice more health benefits from fast rather than weight loss, then there are some fast that works better when compared to other options. Be aware, even though all fasts will help you lose weight and live a healthier life, you still need to make sure that you are following the plan which is right for your needs.

The 12 hours fast

Fasting for 12 hours, is one of the ways to get started with fasting. That is the easiest way to learn how fasting works and to figure out how your body reacts to it. As I previously mentioned before, women tend to find fasting a bit more difficult because of their reproductive systems. Which makes a 12-hour fast an excellent tool for women to find out how their body reacts, and to slowly start to control their hunger cravings.

The 12-hour fast is very simple to follow, and you will be fasting for half the day and eating for half the day. When I put it like that, it doesn't sound so bad, does it? Although a 12-hour fast is still considered a fast and you will see some benefits from it, it won't be as drastic as something like a 16 hour fast or anything along that line. The 12-hour fast works are great to get your body to prepare for more extended fasting and to show you what fasting feels like; it is merely a beginner's tool.

Nonetheless, we highly recommend 12-hour fast for women who are just starting intermittent fasting. The best way to go about 12 hours fast would be to eat from 8 am till 8 pm and then from 8 pm to 8 am not eat anything at all, even though this might sound easy for some it will still catch up on you. We recommend you follow the 12-hour fast for four weeks or until you feel like you can fast for a more extended period of time. But, most of the time, four weeks does the trick for beginners.

Even though studies are showing that 12-hour fast tends to be the perfect time for fasting as tested on rats.

It is still recommended that you fast for a little bit of more extended time, as from personal experience and speaking with other experts in the field of intermittent fasting they recommend ideal fast should be 16 to 20 hours. Regardless when you fast for 12 hours, you'll start to see benefits such as your insulin sensitivity going up your fat loss will kick up a notch, and you will notice more mental focus.

The 12-hour fast does everything right, which makes the 12 hours fast a jack of all trades but a master of none. It is recommended that you only follow this method for a short period to see some results and to get used to fasting, you can pick any time frame you want to fast during. As we previously mentioned before, you can eat from 8 am to 8 pm and not eat from 8 pm to 8 am the next day. The timings won't make a drastic difference in the type of results you will be getting from the 12 hours fast. As long as you pick a time that works for you, then you should be good.

16 Hour fast

This is the fasting method, which has been popularized to be intermittent fasting. Many people use this method to lose weight and to gain some muscle, especially men. But the 16-hour fast has been used successfully by women as well, Martin Bekhan who popularized this method truly lives by it. He has noticed the better fat loss, better health, and more muscle mass by following this plan. Now if putting on muscle is not your goal, the 16-hour fast still has some things to consider.

Most people notice when they start 16 hours fast, is the ability to lose body fat without counting any calories or eating any specific foods. Since the 8-hour window becomes too short of overeating, followers of the 16/8 intermittent fasting method tend to see amazing results in the weight loss department. From my personal experience, I can say that 16 by eight was one of the best ways to lose fat, very easy to follow and 16 hours of fasting is not so hard, overall the results were tremendous. On top of losing weight, I noticed that my skin started to look a lot better, which was precisely what I was looking for.

In one of the newer studies done on obese individuals, they noticed not only fat loss but also reduction and blood pressure. Which means 16/8 method is excellent for fat loss and lowering the risk of cardiovascular diseases and heart diseases, even though this study was taken part on obese people it is still great to have been backed up by science. Bumping up from 12 hours to 16 hours, you will not notice a big difference in insulin sensitivity and mental focus. But you will see more benefits towards that cellular rejuvenation and better results in fat loss.

You will also notice more detox benefits from the 16 hours fast if compared to the 12 hours, which makes the 16-hour fast a lot more similar to the 12 hours fast. Think of the 16 hours fast as the full version of intermittent fasting whereas the 12-hour fast is the trial version, even though there is only 4-hour difference between the two it stills makes up for a drastic change.

Once you start fasting for 16 hours instead of 12, you will notice better fat loss and more health benefits from it. Just like the 12 hours fast, you can follow whichever way you want to pursue this fasting, the timings can be based on your lifestyle. We recommend fasting from 10 pm to 2 pm and eat from 2 pm to 10 pm, but make sure to pick a time that works for you.

Fast for 2 days per week

This fasting method was popularized by Michael Mosley, who is a doctor and journalist. Since this method has no studies to prove its benefits, it is still a method used by many people. Even though this method does not have any reliable research to back it up, benefits which are stated include better brain function, Reducing the risk of heart disease, stroke, cancer, and improving cholesterol levels.

This method can get tough to follow for some people. However, it will put you in a twenty percent calorie deficit, which is a great place to be in if your goal is to lose body fat. This could be an excellent way to lose excess body fat if you can handle it, on that note, let's talk about this method and how it works.

 Also known as the 5:2 method, is where the person eats an average amount of calories throughout the week and restricts their calories to five hundred/six hundred calories a day for two days. The guideline suggests five hundred calories a day for women and six hundred calories for men on fasting days. The method recommends you have two meals divided into your calories for the day when fasting, which means two meals of two fifty calories for women and two meals of three hundred calories a day for men.

Your calories will not be completely cut out throughout those two days, so make sure you are drinking a ton of water and other no-calorie liquids in between your meals on fasting days. Now the best way that you can go about using this method of fasting would generally be eating thru Monday to Friday then fasting over the weekend, and my recommendation would be fast when you don't have work or if you are doing anything physically demanding like working out.

This will ensure you don't feel tired or worst go hypoglycemic as you will be "fasting" for a very long time, so make sure you are fasting on days you are not working or doing anything physically demanding. Also, the great thing about this method is that there is no food restriction during non-fasting days, which is a good thing for some you foodies out there. Now there are some benefits to these methods, and let us talk about that.

The primary benefit is that you will lose body fat and that too quite quickly, as a result of eating so little during those two days of fasting. I have personally followed this plan just as an experiment, and I have to say, and I did lose body fat in those two weeks, which I followed it. If your goal is fat loss without restricting your diet as much, then this method can be the one for you.

Another benefit claimed are lower cholesterol, lower risk of heart disease and cancer, which is fantastic for everyone following this method of fasting. But then again, these benefits are claimed, not proven so don't follow this method if your goal is to lower the risk of diseases there are other fasting methods in this book that you can follow to get those benefits. The great thing about this fasting method is that you will get to eat what you want to eat, no need to restrict yourself on non-fasting days, but if I were you, I would still be careful. Not to overeat if your goal is to lose body fat, so those are the benefits now let's talk about the cons. This method is not ideal by any means, there are some flaws to this method, and one of them was used in a positive, but it is being used in con. In this method, you can eat whatever you want to eat, which is a flaw since people will eat a ton of junk food as an excuse and not do any justice to their health. I believe that fasting should be accompanied with a well-balanced, healthy diet and having junk food on occasion, so I don't like the fact of having whatever you want on your non-fasting days as it can take away from the benefits of fasting.

Another flaw of this method is that it can be tough for some people to make it a lifestyle as fasting for two days straight can be a problem, but if it works for you then go for it. The main flaw is that there so no backing up the claims that this method is claiming. Although this is a fasting method and fasting has a lot of benefits which have been backed up, this method doesn't so as I said before don't follow this diet if your sole purpose is to lower the risk of diseases. If you follow a workout plan that requires strength training, then this fasting method might not be the one for you, as this method can hinder your workout quality as it did for some people.

So now you know all about the 5:2 method, this method can be used with great success if your goal is to lose body fat and have no restrictions to your diet on non-fasting days. But please use this method for the right reasons, don't use it if you want a lowered risk of diseases as studies have not proved it.

Other fasting methods can be followed if your goal is lower the risks, and if your goal is to get stronger and put on some muscle then this method won't be ideal as this method can affect your workouts. All in all, if this method is being used for the right reasons, then it can lead you into great success in weight loss goals. If this method matches your lifestyle and goals, then follow this fasting protocol. But our recommendation would be to use this plan with a grain of salt and to only use for a short period. As we don't think this method is a sustainable fasting protocol like the 16/8.

Alternate day fasting

Very similar to the two days a week fasting, this method requires you usually eat on one day and the next day fast. For the fasting period, you are allowed to have 500 calories a day for women and 600 calories for men. However, you can take it up a notch and not eat any calories at all, which is not recommended by most but done by some. The whole reason behind the alternative fasting was to help people lose weight quickly; people have seen similar results as the 5:2 method where they lose a lot of body fat fast. This method has also been shown to lower the risk of diabetes, which is a great plus for people looking to lose weight and reduces the risk of diabetes.

This method allows you typically to fast three days in a week, putting you at a 25% caloric deficit, which is a little bit more than the 5:2 method. What I like about this fasting method is the frequency. If compared to the 5:2 method, you are fasting more frequently and more regularly. Whereas in the 5:2 method you are eating whatever you want for five days, and then fasting for two whole days straight, this makes it a little bit more reputable for me.

That being said, the same cons follow for this one. On your fasting days, you aren't genuinely fasting, and you can if you decide to but it not healthy, especially for women to fast for 24 hours so frequently. Another disadvantage of this diet would be the allowance of eating whatever they want, although it is excellent for people who like to eat junk food, it is not so healthy, especially on fasting days. Most people will eat something non-dense like a slice of pizza, whereas you should be eating more of a dense meal to see better health changes overall.

Which makes this diet an excellent tool for weight loss, since it will help keep in a caloric deficit throughout the week. However, this diet is not a great way to see some health benefits from, making it very similar to the 5:2 fasting method. One great thing about this method when compared to the 5:2 method, is the ability to maintain strength during workouts. Since your fast will be very cyclical, your chances of losing a lot of strength will be lower, which makes this diet ideal for someone looking to lose fat and maintain a healthy strength level thru out.

Finally, make sure that if you decide to follow this fasting protocol, it is for the right reasons. If you want to lose weight quickly and you have a comfortable going lifestyle, then this plan might be the answer for you. Also, just like the 5:2 method, I would not recommend you follow this fasting method for a prolonged period of time as it can be unhealthy. However, besides all the negatives of this fasting protocol, there are a ton of positives, especially if you are looking to lose weight.

Weekly 24 hour fast

The 24 hours fast has been used widely by many fitness professionals out there. Brad Pilon, the author of eat stop eat once, said: "prolonged calories restriction is the only way to fat loss." Which is the reason why the weekly 24 hours fast was created, easy as it sounds once a week you eat no calories. After you have completed the fast, eat regularly as you would if you were not fasting.

The whole premises behind this fasting protocol is to put you in a caloric deficit. For example, if you require 2,500 calories to maintain your weight, then eat 2,500 calories a day but fast for one of those days. The claims of the weekly fasting method are, weight loss lowered the risk of diseases such as diabetes and many others. Unfortunately, in the weekly 24 hours fasts, the claims haven't been backed up with science. However, this fasting protocol has shown to speed up weight loss.

Many followers of this fasting protocol have seen fantastic weight loss effects, which makes this a tremendous tool for fat loss, also really good for detoxing your body. The 24-hour fast will help you get rid of any toxins in your intestines and other organs, believe it or not digesting food is a hard task for our body. Not giving your intestines and other organs a break from digesting can lead to poor digestion, this is where the weekly 24-hour fasting shines. People who follow this fast, have noticed better digestion and healthier hair and skin because of cell rejuvenation effects it has.

The weekly 24 hours fast has shown to help with cell rejuvenation or also known as autophagy, which makes this protocol great for followers looking to lose weight and see results like better digestion and cell rejuvenation. Even though this protocol comes with a host of benefits, there are still some concerns. Even though you are fasting for only one day a week, 24 hours fast can become very hard for some, especially women, because of the hunger craving.

It would be best if you had a great support system to pull through the 24 hours fast, another fallback of this fast would be the post-binge eating cravings. Many followers have noticed insane amounts of food craving the day after fasting if you overeat throughout the week and fast for only one day, the chances of you losing weight will be slim to none. Make sure you have the will power to avoid these food cravings once you get them, as indulging in them would not be great if you are looking to lose body fat.

In conclusion, this protocol is ideal for people who have fasted for an extended period of time before. We would not recommend this fasting protocol to an absolute beginner, as it can be tough to follow through. Fasting has no benefit if you can't follow thru, so make sure you pick the right one.

Meal Skipping

This method is something people used to their body prepared for fasting, now to be clear I don't consider this to be as beneficial as most fasting protocol, and I repeat I don't believe this method to be as helpful as most fasting protocol. Now saying that would I recommend this method to someone else? The answer is yes! Why you ask, the simple reason this method is one of the easiest to follow, and it prepares you for fasting methods that will help you with better physical health and wellness. Would I recommend someone make this method their lifestyle, and the answer would be no.

Only consider this if you have never followed a fasting method before and you want to slowly build up to a longer fast, which would make this method the one for you. Some readers can completely ignore this method and start with other fasting method's listed above, if you have experience fasting before for fifteen days then you should be able to follow a more "intense" protocols. None the less, let's talk about this method. The whole point of this method is for you to start skipping meals, in between the day to ease you into a longer fast.

So what you can do if you decide to follow this plan is to start by skipping breakfast then have some lunch and dinner, slowly building up to a longer fast. If you want, you can even have a snack instead of skipping breakfast, which will make it easier for you. The whole point is to make you feel comfortable before taking the big step, and this method allows you to take baby steps into the great realm of fasting. Which I think is the plus of this fasting method.

There are some benefits to this type of fasting method. One of the things that you might notice, especially starting is that you will most likely lose some fat. Often, we don't realize how much we overeat, and the average person tends to eat more than he or she should. Most North American diet consists of foods which are loaded with carbohydrates, sugar, and a ton of "bad fat" such as trans fat in their diet, which leads to most of the obesity issues in our society. One meal on average tends to be six hundred to a thousand calories per meal.

Now if you skip one meal every day for a week, you are looking to cut about forty two-hundred to seven thousand calories a week, a pound of fat has thirty-five-hundred calories so you can defiantly see some fat loss benefits. This method will also give your gut a break from digesting all this processed food that some readers might be eating, which means better gut health overall. You can see all the benefits of this method, but this fasting method is something that you should not use as a protocol to lose fat in the long term as it can leave you malnourished in the end.

See our primary goal with this book is to show you how to live a healthy life both physically and mentally, sometimes our body gives us signals to skip meals and without even knowing you would skip a meal just because you felt like it. We are always using this method, but then the next day instead of three, we have four meals and not to mention a big and unhealthy one. So our body always makes us clean our gut time to time organically, one thing people can get carried away within this method is since they skip a meal, they think they can have anything their heart desires.

Which should not be the case, in my opinion, you need to be eating healthy doesn't matter if you choose to fast or not if you want to be free of health complications in future and looking good. By eating healthy we make sure to get all our micronutrients in, like our vitamins and minerals for the day and your macronutrients like your calories, fats, carbs and protein depending on your fitness and aesthetic goals.

Another thing that should not be left out is the consumption of water if you can't seem to skip the meal, and you tend to get hungry, drink more water during your fast. Not only will that hydrate you, but it will also get rid of toxins in your body and help you with fat loss if that's your goal. At the end of the day, if you want to ease into this fasting lifestyle, you should use this method as a tool to get you up to a longer fast, so you don't fall off track. Just make sure you are using it for the right reasons if 12 hours soon is too much for you to begin with, then consider this protocol and move up from there.

The warrior diet

This method is more based on our ancestors' eating habits. Created by Ori Hofmekler, this method suggests us to "eat like a warrior." In the earlier times fasting thru out the day and only having a four-hour window to eat a big meal was a norm for us humans, as Hofmekler thinks human were created to eat like this. This method was based on his belief system and how humans should be eating instead of using science-based evidence and studies. In this method you are allowed to have mostly whatever you want in that four-hour eating window, go by what you feel and also don't go by macronutrient count eat how much ever you want to eat.

Another thing which is advocated in this method is that you will be more suited for burning fat for energy, claimed by Ori Hofmekler. If you follow this diet, you will lose body fat and won't have to count calories. So in this method, you have to fast for twenty hours and have an eating window of only four hours.

Now if you are currently using the "16/8" method then switching up to the warrior diet won't be such a shock to your body, but if you are going to go from an average eating habit to this, then I will be hard for you physically. I would recommend starting with fasting for twelve hours and slowly building up to the twenty-hour mark. If fasting for twelve hours can get challenging for you, then I would suggest slowly skipping meals like breakfast, and then when that feels easy slowly skipping breakfast and lunch until you get to the point where you can fast for twenty hours of the day.

Now, the way it is recommended to follow this method is to fast in the day time and eat at the night time, as warriors would do after hunting and preparing their meals at the end of the day. You can have your meals at any time even before going to bed, and this diet should be followed just like the ancient times like the warrior did, meaning fast in the morning and feast at night. In this diet, you can have fruits and vegetables, but it's recommended you stay away from canned fruits and vegetables, also their juices.

In this method, it's highly recommended to workout in an empty stomach, to stimulate a warrior lifestyle. It is suggested to work out for thirty to forty-five minutes of intense workouts, with the use of compound movements like pull-ups, push-ups, and squats, which use more than one muscle group. You can still consume water, and other non-calorie drinks, so don't be scared to workout not hydrated.

So in conclusion, this diet is based on a lifestyle which warriors had back in ancient times, which was a selling factor for some people, including me. Since this diet has no science or studies to back it up, it can be a turn off to some people when it comes to following a fasting protocol since they might want to see health benefits like lowering the risk of diabetes and other things of that nature.

Even though this method is quite similar to "16/8", I think it should help lower risk of diseases but then again, no research on it. On the other hand, if your goal is to feel and look like a warrior, this method will be the right one for you. Although I haven't followed this plan long enough to see drastic physical changes, I have met people who have completely transformed their physical appearance and health also their energy levels have drastically changed for the better. This method has resulted in success for most people, and when I followed it for one week, I felt like "16-8" is ideal for me as I was feeling the same on this method.

One thing I didn't like about this method is that you have to work out on an empty stomach, as with "16/8" I would workout fed. So if you don't mind working out on an empty stomach and you want to live a warrior lifestyle, then this method might be for you.

Even though this goes with no saying, always get recommended by your doctor before you follow this method or another method listed in this book. This method can be pretty hard for you in the beginning; make sure you don't go into it without easing into fasting. I hope you see the results that you are looking for following this fasting method.

We have now gone thru all the fasting methods, and you might have learned a lot from this chapter. Many people might say that fasting works differently on men as compared to women, but besides the hunger portion, it is the same. As long as you follow these fasts safety and with the guidance of your doctor, you should be fine.

Also, if you read these chapters carefully, you might have noticed that some fasts are suited better for specific results. Even though all fasts will help you achieve fat loss and overall health benefits, there are some protocols tailored for weight loss and others which are suited for whole, healthy well-being.

When you are picking out which fasting protocol to follow, consider lifestyle, and your goals as most of them will fit your needs. Overall know what you want out of intermittent fasting. Also, if you pick the right fasting protocol, then you should see the benefits which you have been looking to get.

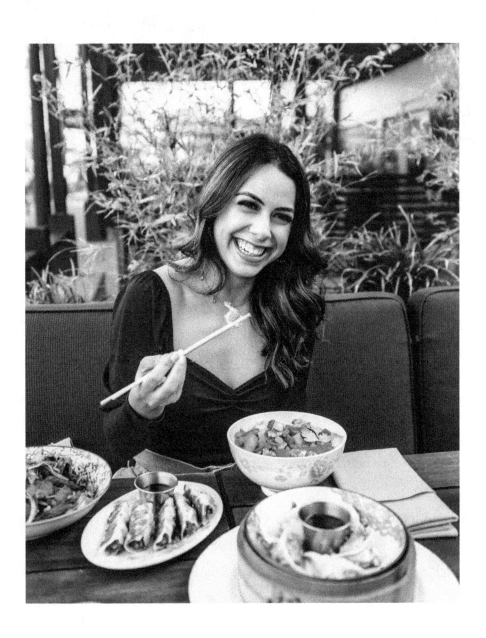

Chapter 4: Intermittent Fasting and Women

As we mentioned to you previously, intermittent fasting does not yield drastically different results in both men and women. However, there are many differences in regards to how women should follow intermittent fasting. The great news is that women can take part in all the fast's listed in this book, regardless we need to talk about intermittent fasting for women.

Some claims are suggesting that intermittent fasting needs to be modified, which is true to a certain degree if women use the easier going fasting protocols, which are available to review in the previous chapters. Then they should have no problem with intermittent fasting, and the problems start to occur when 48 hours+ fasts begin to take place.

Nonetheless, you should know the claims and studies done on women in regards to intermittent fasting. There was one study suggesting that blood sugar worsened in women after three weeks of intermittent fasting. Moreover, many sources are claiming that changes in women menstrual cycle will occur. As we explained before, because of women reproductive system, they are susceptible to lower calories.

Hence, making people believe that women do not indulge in intermittent fasting, which we don't agree. If done tastefully, intermittent fasting has resulted in excellent health and weight loss benefits for women. So in this chapter, we will go thru exactly how intermittent fasting effects women in all aspects, such as hormones, hunger craving, and many more things are on the agenda. With that in mind, let's get into the nitty-gritty.

The key to intermittent fasting for women in autophagy

You might have heard of autophagy in this book so far, now let me explain to you what autophagy truly means. Autophagy is a biological process which comes from the Greek word "auto," meaning "self" and "phagy," meaning "eat." It is a process where our body cleans out the bad cells and replace them with newer healthy ones, which is excellent for anyone looking to live a healthier life.

But sometimes, our body cannot get this process going for hosts of reasons. Manly because we eat the food we can't digest properly, which makes our body work extra hard to cope up with the food instead of getting rid of "bad cells." As we get older, the process becomes less efficient. One of the proven ways to fix this issue, especially for women is by fasting for 12 or more hours and allowing your body to focus more on getting rid of the "bad cells," by replacing them with newer and stronger ones.

This method works exceptionally well, especially on women, to rejuvenate their cells and to see the health benefits. The great news about autophagy is that you don't need to fast for an indefinite amount of time to notice the results, 12 to 16 hours of fast will do. Which means women don't need to put yourself at risk by fasting for a prolonged period; this makes intermittent fasting a tool for women looking to stay young for more extended periods.

Remember that autophagy should not be just for anti-aging purposes, as it can help you with hosts of things. Consider autophagy as a detox for your whole body, and believe it or not most people need it. Forget cleansing diets, and if you truly want to detox your body, then you need to fast for at least 12 hours a day.

For women, 12-16 hours should not result in adverse effects. You will also reduce the risk of cancer because you will have newer and stronger cells at your disposal; another great benefit would be the fact that your metabolism will go up helping you with weight loss.

All in all, promoting the process of autophagy a great way to encourage better health, especially for women. Having healthier cells in a women's body will help you by having a better reproductive system, and you will have a higher chance of conceiving. Even though these claims haven't been backed up, it is still good to know that some excellent benefits come with intermittent fasting for women.

Finally, you will notice benefits such as better skin, better digestion more energy throughout the day. To see the best results, fast for 12 to 16 hours a day, three times a week. Make sure you space out your days, instead of doing all the fasts back to back. If you want to fast through the week as many do, then make sure not to prolong it for more than 6-8 weeks.

Fasting and female hormones

Intermittent fasting has shown to affect females' hormones, and there are some things women need to consider before they start fasting. Some studies are showing how intermittent fasting can negatively impact the female's reproductive system, and the reason why these shifts occur is that women are sensitive to lower calorie intake. When the calories are low for women, a small part of the brain known as the hypothalamus is affected.

Hypothalamus can disrupt the production of gonadotropin-releasing hormone (GnRH), which is responsible for releasing the two reproductive hormones, luteinizing hormone (LH) and follicle stimulating hormone (FSH). Once these hormones have been affected negatively from an extended period by restricting calories, you will be running a risk of irregular periods, infertility, poor bone health, and other health risks. Even though autophagy has shown to do the opposite, it puts women in a complicated situation when it comes to fasting. For that reason, we don't recommend women fast for more than 24 hours as it can affect women hormone in a very drastic manner.

Instead, women should use a modified approach that we talked about in this book. To make sure women don't notice any hormone imbalance, fast alternate days instead of back to back, keeping you in a safe place. If you want to fast aggressively for weight loss, then our recommendation is not to prolong it for more than 4-6 weeks. But then again, make sure you consult a professional before you may start fasting as everybody is different. On the plus side, there are many benefits women will notice if they begin fasting the right way. As we know, heart disease is killing people every day, in one study done on obese women showed that intermittent fasting lowered LDL cholesterol or which is the leading cause of heart problems in North America.

Also, intermittent fasting has shown to make you more insulin sensitive. In one study of 100 obese women showed that six months of intermittent fasting reduced insulin levels by 29% and insulin resistance by 19 %, although blood sugar remained the same. Having higher sensitively to insulin has shown to lower the risk of type 2 diabetes, but intermittent fasting may not be beneficial for women as it is for men in regards to blood sugar. In mice, it has been shown to increase the longevity by 33% although long term studies on humans are yet to be determined.

Finally, intermittent fasting can reduce inflammation levels. Even though more studies need to be executed for women and intermittent fasting, it is pretty clear that there are hosts of benefits if done right. As long as you are taking intermittent fasting the right way, and you are not abusing it, your hormones should be in check. Remember, if you are pregnant, this might affect you very differently. Moreover, we do not recommend women fast when they are pregnant or trying to conceive, but as long as you know the repercussions of fasting too long.

Why intermittent fasting effects women's hormone more than men's?

If you have been doing research online, then you might have read claims such as "intermittent fasting is not for women" or "if women intermittent fast, their hormones will be out of whack." Which isn't the case, as we will discuss how intermittent fasting truly affects women's hormone as when compared to men.

To briefly talk about men, they were created to "hunt and gather" so to speak. Unlike women, they do not have to carry a baby, which is one of the reasons why intermittent fasting does not affect men as drastically as women. Women are more susceptive to hormones which are related to hunger, and the reason behind is women's reproductive system as previously mentioned.

The good news is, it will not affect your thyroid as some "experts" will claim, women recognize hunger at a higher degree than men. We recently talked about the Hypothalamus gonadotropin-releasing hormone (GnRH), luteinizing hormone (LH) and follicle stimulating hormone (FSH), which is responsible for making testosterone and sperm in men and triggering estrogen and ovulation in women.

Women tend to trigger these hormones differently when compared to men, and the main problem occurs because of kisspeptin. For readers that don't know what kisspeptin is, it is a protein like molecules that neurons use to communicate with each other. Women tend to produce more kisspeptin when compared to men, which is a precursor to (GnRH).

As you know (GnRH) is going to dictate how women produce estrogen and how men are going to produce testosterone; another thing is that kisspeptin is very sensitive to the hunger hormone. If you remember, we mentioned that women are more vulnerable to the hunger hormone when compared to men? The reason behind is kisspeptin, which causes women to produce less kisspeptin and leads to lower progesterone. In one study done on rats, showed that when female rats fast for one day which is more like a week for women, it caused them to lose 19% of their body weight but their ovaries shrunk significantly.

Also, they noticed that female rats luteinizing hormone plummeted, and their estrogen levels went thru the roof. To briefly touch upon thyroid, t3 levels were deceased. But, t3 levels are always decreasing between meals. The t4 which is responsible for producing thyroid remained the same, which means the thyroid isn't being affected drastically. It is always suggested that you get regular blood work done to ensure your thyroid is fine, but one of them to tell if it isn't is by seeing how could you get.

If you feel cold all the time, then the chances are your thyroid is lower. If you notice that you are getting starving throughout the day, and it becomes tough to fast, then break the fast and try it again later. As women, you need to listen to your more than men, as women tend to be more sensitive to hormones when intermittent fasting.

Eating enough calories

Since you now know the science behind intermittent fasting and how it can affect women's hormone, let us talk about eating enough calories, especially for women. Believe it or not, this is an important topic to discuss. Especially for women who are much more sensitive to hunger hormones or hormones in general when compared to men. Even though you might be fasting for weight loss, it is critical that you enough calories support your bodily function as a woman. Ideally speaking women who are trying to lose weight should not eat bellow 200 calories of their maintenance, calculating your maintenance calories the formula is (bodyweight x 12).

Meaning, if your maintenance calories are 2,000 and you are looking to lose weight, then you should not cut it down less than 1,800. If you are someone looking to lose weight with intermittent fasting, we recommend having a macronutrient break down of 20% carbs 50% protein and 30% fats; this shows the percentage of calories coming from specific macronutrients.

We are keeping the carbs low to prevent insulin spikes in check if you are looking to lose weight, we want to keep the insulin as flatlined as possible. However, if you are someone looking to maintain weight and reap the health benefits of intermittent fasting, then we recommend having a macronutrient breakdown of 30% carbs 40% protein 30% fats since we have covered the calorie intake, lets briefly talk about the types of food you should be eating. What you eat to break your fast is just as essential as the number of calories you should be consuming. One thing you need to understand is not to go overboard on the fasting.

As you know, carbs tend to spike your insulin, and when you're fasting, your insulin levels are low, meaning whatever you eat, your body will be sensitive to it. Having spikes of insulin slows down fat loss. Therefore, lower insulin equals more fat burning. If you break your fast with higher amounts of carbs, you will be shutting down the fat burning process. Instead, what we recommend is eating two meals when you break in your eating window. The first one should be lower in carbs and higher in fats and protein; this will ensure you don't turn off your fat burning and get the most out of your fast. The second meal could be higher carbs, and this will help you get ready for the next day if you are fasting.

Another to remember is that your gut will be susceptible to high acidic foods such and drinks, so make sure you stick to foods which are less acidic when you break your fast. Greek yogurt, chicken with some veggies or even soup works great to break your fast. Now whether your goal is to lose weight or live a healthier life, it is essential that you follow the right calorie intake and macronutrients intake. These tips will go a long way with both the criteria listed.

How to avoid feeling underfed
Since you now know how much to eat, let's talk about how to prevent feeling underfed. Believe it or not, both men and women notice this problem, which causes them to overeat. We need to make sure you don't

feed underfed to avoid things like breaking a fast too soon or overeating. There is a couple of technique we can provide you with that shall help you with the feeling of underfed.

The first technique we recommend would be eating wholesome, healthy foods which have a lot of fiber in them. Even though you are free to eat whatever you want, it is still not recommended that you eat unhealthily. When you break you're fast, the food you should be eating is high fiber lower carbs and moderate protein. What the fiber will do is help you feel fuller through the day, making you feel less underfed.

An example of this would be to eat more green leafy vegetables, as they will make you feel fuller for a long time. Since we are on the topic of plants, let us talk about vitamins, you need to have micronutrients dense meals when you are fasting. If you are feeling underfed when fasting, the chances are that you are not consuming enough vitamins and minerals, making you feel underfed.

Make sure you are getting your daily mineral intake during your eating window to avoid such adverse effects; you could take a vitamin supplement during your fasting window to obtain your minerals. But don't use the supplement to take care of your vitamin needs, make sure you are eating healthy foods instead of junk food to feel thoroughly fed. Also, drinking water for the whole day is essential. If you are not drinking enough water, then you have a much higher chance of feeling underfed.

Not only will the water help you feel fuller, but it will also help you to get rid of toxins in your body. Water is a must for better fasting experience; another thing which can curb your hunger is coffee. If you drink black coffee during your fast, it will help you control any hunger cravings you might be having which will make you feel less underfed.

One recommendation would be drinking your coffee during the earlier times of the day, instead of later. As drinking coffee then makes you crash pretty hard, which will make you crave more, so make sure you stay away from coffee later during the day. Perhaps consume your coffee earlier in the morning or before your workout works the best, but the main take away would be not to consume junk. Even though fasting allows you to eat whatever you want, it doesn't mean you should, as it can lead you feeling underfed and hungry in the long run. Make sure you are following all these steps to ensure not handling underfed, and as you know, women tend to experience more hunger.

How often should women follow intermittent fasting

When it comes to fasting, women are more sensitive than men. Hence, making the timings and the duration of fasting a bit more restricted than men. Experts suggest that women should have a more relaxed approach than men. This may include shorter fasting days, lesser fasting days, and sometimes eating some food during the fast. We always recommend women to not fast longer than 24 hours, that's why all the fasting protocols listed in this book have a fasting window of no more than 24 hours.

Also, whichever fasting protocol you decide to choose, make sure it is sustainable to you. As it can lead to fewer results overall and disappointment, these being the surface level issues. If women fast for longer than 24 hours, it can lead to hormones going out of whack, and you what could happen then. Another thing to make sure of would be to fast consecutive days in the beginning, and it is recommended that women fast three times a week on consecutive days to ensure they can handle it.

Follow this protocol for the first three weeks, and eventually, if your physician gives you the go, then start lasting longer. With that being said, some women should not follow intermittent fasting. If you are pregnant, trying to conceive, nursing, or under chronic stress, then fasting should not be done. This now brings me to the period women should fast for. Ideally, women should follow a fasting protocol for no longer than eight weeks.

It is ideal for women to take a break from internment fasting after fasting for eight weeks, women should take a whole week off from fasting ideally two weeks off. If you start to notice symptoms such as irregular period, metabolic stress, anxiety, depression, and insomnia, then stop fasting right away and speak with your doctor. These could be a sign of fasting for too long, so make sure you are looking out for these symptoms every time. There are some fasts you should not do for a prolonged period, such as the 5:2 method and the alternate day fasting.

For these two fasting protocols makes sure you are not exceeding the six-week mark of following it. Finally, women need to stay on alert when they are fasting, know your body, and make sure you feel right and healthy when you are fasting. Some hunger cravings are fine, but if you start to notice insanity high food cravings which you can't control no matter what, then it is safer to eat some food rather than put your hormones and body in danger.

Fasting can be very fragile in terms of improving health or deteriorating it, especially in women. Which means you need to make sure you ease into fasting and to take regular breaks from it. The timelines we recommend in this chapter works for most women, but consult with a professional before you start or stop a fasting protocol! Good luck.

Symptoms you should look out for

There are many signs to look for when intermittent fasting since you know most of the things related to intermittent fasting by now, let's talk about the significant symptoms to look out. The first one being hunger, many followers of intermittent fasting will notice insane amounts of desire when following intermittent fasting. Which is a given, since you will be going from eating four to six meals throughout the day to none.

The first couple of days will require a ton of willpower to get thru, but eventually, it will subside and get better in a week. Give it some time for your body to get used to intermittent fasting, and be aware of the fact that it will be a shock in the beginning. Besides hunger, cravings for food is very evident when following intermittent fasting. Chances of you breaking your fast will be very high, especially when you are just getting started with it. You will crave foods like a candy bar, fruits, soda's anything which will give you a ton of sugar quickly. You will have to fight these cravings as they will kick in so make sure you don't indulge in them, Headaches is another thing which beginners might notice.

When you start your intermittent fasting, you will see symptoms such as headaches, don't get worried as they will subside in a week in most cases. Make sure you are drinking plenty of water during your fasting window and after, as this will make it easy for your body to cope with the headaches.

One of the main symptoms you should be looking out for would be feeling cold. You will be contacting cold for the first week, but if it continues past the three-week mark then consider modifying your fasting protocol. Intermittent fasting has shown to increase blood flow to your fat stores for your body to use it for energy, but if you start feeling cold shivering past the three-week mark, then it is a symptom you should be looking out.

Since you will be drinking a lot of water, this will make you feel even colder through the day so unless you feel cold, don't take it seriously. Speaking of drinking water, you will also notice you going to the bathroom a lot. It is because of your water consumption, and there isn't a way around it since we don't recommend you drink less water. These are the main symptoms you will notice when you first start intermittent fasting, and they usually last three weeks.

If you experience these symptoms at the same magnitude as you were the first week, then please modify your fasting protocol as it might not be suitable for your body. If you healthily want to follow intermittent fasting, then it is best to look out for these symptoms and to listen to your body. If you're going to avoid these symptoms, then ease into intermittent fasting and making sure it isn't a shock for your body from the get-go.

Tips for intermittent fasting for women

Let's talk about some quick tips women need to consider before they start intermittent fasting, as there are some great ones to find before you start. The first tip would be to drink a ton of water when fasting, pretty easy to follow and understand. You need to drink water to curb your cravings, as you know, women tend to crave foods more than men do only because of the hormone response.

Drinking water will also help you control the headache symptoms you might get, overall drinking water is a must. Drinking tea and coffee will help you manage your hunger throughout the day; it will also give you more energy in the beginning stages of fasting.

Just make sure you drink black coffee or black/green tea, don't add any sugar or milk as it will break your fast if you do that. If you find yourself around people who aren't supportive of your fasting endeavors, then make sure you stay away from them or at least avoid talking about fasting. The last thing you want is unsupportive people when you are following intermittent fasting, so make sure you stay away from them and stay positive. Finally, give yourself at least a month when you start intermittent fasting.

Many people don't realize that it will take some time to start seeing changes in their body; four weeks is a good time for your body to begin adapting to intermittent fasting. Meaning, you need to keep up the fast for at least a month for you to make a judgment whether fasting is for you or not, and most of the time it works out in your favor. In the first four weeks of fasting, you will notice hunger waves avoid them by drinking coffee or tea. The main tip when intermittent fasting would be to not binge eat, when you break your fast you will have the craving to binge eat.

Avoid it, follow our macros and eating patterns which we have listed above in this chapter. If you want to develop your eating pattern that's fine as well, make sure not a lot of carbs are on your plate in your first meal as this will make you binge eat later. Making sure you don't overeat is essential for intermittent fasting, as it will dictate your goals. If you are looking to lose weight, then make sure you eat portion-controlled meals instead of eating whatever your heart desires. These are all the primary tips, make sure you follow them, so you don't end up giving up too soon.

All in all, these tips will help you in the future. As you will see how much easier fasting becomes for you once you start considering these tips, but don't forget to listen to your body as we previously mentioned. Looking out for your health first is very important, so if you feel like these tips are not helping you within three weeks, then modify your fasting.

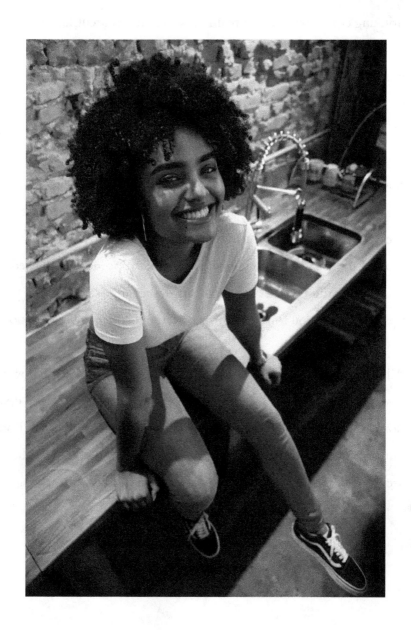

Chapter 5: Hormones

In this chapter, we are going to be talking about hormonal changes that you might see when following intermittent fasting. As we have briefly talked about intermittent fasting, and what it can do for you when it comes to hormonal changes. We will get into depth when it comes to the hormonal changes and what intermittent fasting can do for women. It is important that we understand this topic as it will dictate how well your fast will go or won't go, and the benefits you will be able to see you from it. The first thing you need to keep in mind is that intermittent fasting is very different for both men and women, as you can tell by reading this book. However, it is essential that you know how different it is and what are the side effects which could happen when following intermittent fasting and the hormonal changes. Most of the time, the difference is only hormonal.

As men and women have different hormones, it is important that you understand them and work on it accordingly. Also, the benefits you might see from intermittent fasting might be different from both men and women, which is also important that we talk about it. The first thing you need to understand would be that intermittent fasting will help you with your insulin sensitivity and for you to help digest food a lot better. Even if you are a man or woman, intermittent fasting will help you with insulin sensitivity. This is very important to understand, as this will help you to prevent diseases such as diabetes and many more. Many people in the North American places are facing diabetes, which is not the greatest disease to have as it can lead to a lot of problems in the long run, which is why intermittent fasting will help you with the hormonal changes and to see better results. Overall, this is one hormonal change which you want as a woman when following intermittent fasting.

There have been studies showing that women tend to get affected more from diabetes than man, which is why intermittent fasting is very crucial to follow when you're a woman and of course to follow it the right way. In conjunction with the insulin sensitivity, intermittent fasting will help to lower your LDL cholesterol. This will help you to fight off any heart diseases which might be present in your family, or if you are facing it. We have briefly talked about it in the previous chapters, but know that intermittent fasting will help you to get rid of diabetes and heart diseases which is significant hormonal change to happen if your goal is to be healthy. Hopefully, that makes sense, let's talk about the hormonal changes that will help you to detoxify your body and see the true benefits of intermittent fasting. As you know, intermittent fasting helps with autophagy, which helps you to rejuvenate yourself.

The way this process works is that it fights off any of the old cells and produces new cells, that are very efficient at functioning. This is one of the hormonal changes, the changes that you should be seeing when following intermittent fasting the right way, and this is one hormonal change that is very crucial for your success when it comes to following intermittent fasting. Another thing intermittent fasting will help you with is that it will lower your hunger hormones, many people don't know this, but if you follow intermittent fasting for a long period, you will feel less hungry throughout the day. What this will help you with is weight loss or fat loss, if your goal is to lose weight and to keep it off for a long period that intermittent fasting is the right answer for you. Not only will this put you in a caloric deficit, but it will help you to not be hungry throughout the whole day. The way it works is that your body will get a custom to not eating for a long time, which will overall help you not to eat unwanted calories and therefore help you to lose weight. Another hormonal change that you might notice when following intermittent fasting would be that your dopamine levels will be a lot higher.

If you guys don't know what dopamine is, it is essentially the feel-good hormone that you feel when you achieve anything. Now, if you're someone looking to be happy for a long period and throughout the day, then make sure that you start following intermittent fasting as it will help you to raise your dopamine levels in your brain and therefore help you feel good. Finally, one of the major hormonal effects that you might see when following intermittent fasting is that your growth hormone will go up even if your woman. This hormone will help you with a lot of things, your sexual hormones and your sleep hormones. This hormone will not only help you to get better sleep but help you perform a lot better in the gym if that's what you're going for. If you're someone looking to enhance your performance at the gym, then make sure that you follow intermittent fasting as it will help you to do so.

All in all, these are all the great benefits with the hormones you will see when following intermittent fasting. Now let's talk about something negative hormonal effects you might see when following intermittent fasting. Believe it or not, there are many side effects that you might see when following intermittent fasting, especially when you are a woman. Since women have to carry a baby for nine months, the hormones are very different than men, which is why you need to make sure you don't affect your hormones when following intermittent fasting. One of the things women have to take care of would be to not over fast. Unlike men, women cannot fast for more than 24 hours as it will result in them permanently damaging their reproductive system. Although any adverse side effects haven't taken place yet, it is important that you'd make sure that you are fasting moderately.

One of the things you need to make sure when following intermittent fasting would be not to follow more than three days in a row. It is advisable that women take one day off from fasting for them to recuperate from all the hormonal effects that would have taken place when fasting, as you read in the previous chapters, we talked about how to fast the right way. Make sure that you read all the chapters and understand what kind of fasting protocol works best for you, and always look out for the symptoms when following intermittent fasting. One of the main symptoms to look out for when following intermittent fasting would be that you feel cold all the time.

If you're following intermittent fasting, do you start to feel cold and nauseous all the time, and chances are it's your hormones telling you that you are under eating severely and that you need to stop fasting as soon as possible. Make sure they understand this topic as clearly as possible; it is important to understand your body and give up when it is time to give up. We talked about this topic in the previous chapters. However, I want to bring it up again so that you understand that it is okay to give up on fasting when you feel like you need to. One of the things you need to make sure when fasting is to not go overboard with it, especially when you're a woman.

Also, make sure that you are eating enough food to feed your body during your eating window. This will help you to stay active, and to keep your body well-fed during intermittent fasting. Keep in mind that you don't have to be in a severe caloric deficit when following intermittent fasting. When you're following intermittent fasting, your insulin sensitivity will be so good that even if you eat a little bit more food you will still have a higher metabolism and you will be burning body fat overall.

Which is one misconception many people have when following intermittent fasting, you have to realize that intermittent fasting does so much to your hormones that you don't even need to be in a big deficit to see results that you have been craving for, which is why intermittent fasting is such a great eating protocol to follow if your goal is to detoxify your body and to see fat loss results. Overall intermittent fasting is not just about losing weight, or to look better, and it will change your hormones in the right way if you follow intermittent fasting correctly. Also, intermittent fasting will help you lose weight even if you are eating a lot of food.

Many people have said that they've lost a lot of weight when following intermittent fasting eating whatever they want. However, we don't recommend that, but then again, many people are claiming that they've lost weight eating whatever they wanted during your eating window. Keep in mind that, you have to follow intermittent fasting the right way if your woman as we have explained to you at length on how to do so. If you understand the basic concept of intermittent fasting and you figure out how to follow it the right way, then there is no stopping you. The hormones will change for the better if you follow this eating protocol the right way. However, it can change for the worst if you don't know how to follow intermittent fasting the correct way. After reading this book, you should have zero issues when it comes to following intermittent fasting the right way, with that being said we are now going to end this chapter thank you so much for sticking till the end.

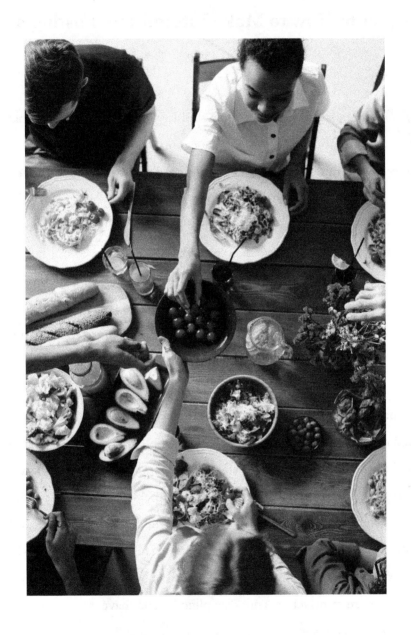

Chapter 6: How to Make Intermittent Fasting a Lifestyle

We will talk about what you should be doing, to make sure that you are not failing in your endeavors to start fasting to live a healthier life overall. This chapter will show you what you could be doing to make fasting your lifestyle and to not only help you to start the Intermittent fasting and stay on track but also to live with this eating plan for the rest of your life. These daily patterns will help you to not fail on your fast, and we understand that you might fail a couple of times in any fasting protocol, and it is understandable to do so. Nonetheless, this chapter will show you how to make sure you are consistent and not failing.

These habits have been followed by many successful people, to get optimal results in all of their aspects of life, whether it be fitness related or anything else. Make sure you start implementing all of these habits after you are done reading this book as it will help you to make fasting your lifestyle. The reason why this chapter might sound philosophical is that the only way you will see success with fasting is if you do it consistently. For you to do that, you need to change your current lifestyle by being more productive and disciplined. You have to remember, healthy eating is more than just a meal; it's a lifestyle.

Plan your day ahead

Planning your day ahead of time is crucial, not only does planning out your day help you be more prepared for your day moving forward, but it will also help you to become more aware of the things you shouldn't be doing, hence wasting your time.

Moreover, planning your day will truly help you with making the most out of your time, that being said, we will talk about two things 1. Benefits of planning out your day 2. How to go about planning out your day. So, without further ado, let us dive into the benefits of planning out your day.

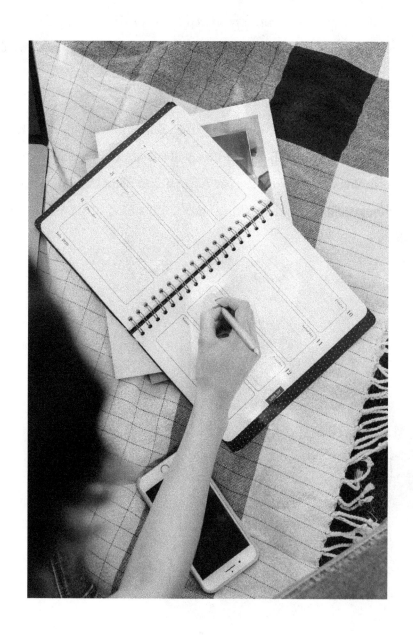

It will help you prioritize:

Yes, planning out your day will help you prioritize a lot of things in your day to day life. You can allow time limits to the things you want to work on the most to least, for example, if you're going to write your book and you are super serious about it. Then you need a specific time limit every day in which you work on a task wholeheartedly without any worries of other things until the time is up. Then you move on to the next job in line, so when you schedule out your whole day, and you give yourself time limits, then you can prioritize your entire day. The same thing goes for your fast, make sure you allocate time for prepping your meals for the next day, which will allow you to have meals ready for you when you need it hence making it easy for you to continue with your fast.

Summarize your normal day:

Now, before we start getting into planning out your whole day ahead, you need to realize that to plan your entire day, you need to know precisely what you are doing that day. Which means you need to write down every single thing you do on a typical day and write down the time you start and end, it needs to be detailed in terms of how long does it take for your transportation to get to work, etc.

Now after you have figured out your whole day, you can decide how to prioritize your day moving on could be cutting out a task that you don't require or shortening your time for a job that doesn't need that much time. After you have your priorities for the day, you can add pleasurable tasks into your day like hanging out with your friends, etc.

Arrange your day:

It is crucial that you arrange your day correctly, so the best way to organize your day is to make sure you get all your essential stuff done earlier in the day when your mind is fresh. After that's done, you can have some time for yourself to relax and do whatever it is that you want. But make sure you get all the things that need to be done before you can move on to free time for yourself. Another thing that will help you is to set time limits on each task, and once you start setting time limits, you will be more likely to get the job done.

Remove all the fluff:

So, what I mean by that is remove all the things that are holding you back from achieving your goals. Make sure you remove all of the things that are holding you back from getting the things that you need to be doing. If you have time for the fluff, do it if not, then work on your priorities first. In conclusion, planning out your day will help you tremendously! Make sure you plan out your day every day to ensure successful and accomplished days.

Stop multitasking

I think we are all guilty of this at a time, and if you are multitasking right now, I need you to stop. Now multitasking could be a lot of things, it could be as small as cooking and texting at the same time, or it could be as big as working on two projects at the same time. Studies are showing how multitasking can reduce your quality of work, which something you don't want to do if your goal is to get the best result out of the thing that you are doing. That being said, there are a lot more reasons as to why you shouldn't be multitasking, so without further ado, lets dive into the primary reasons why multitasking can be harmful.

You're not as productive.

Believe it or not, you tend to be a lot less productive when you are multitasking. When you go from one project to another or anything else for that matter, you don't put all your effort into your work. You are always worried about the project that you will be moving into next. So, moving back and forth from one project to another will affect your productivity if you want to get the most out of your work you need to be focused on one thing at a time and make sure you get it done to the best of your abilities. Plus, you are more likely to make mistakes, which will not help you work at the best of your ability.

You become slower at your work.

When you are multitasking, chances are you will end up being slower at completing your projects. You would be in a better position if you were to focus on one project at a time instead of going back and forth, which of course helps you complete them faster. So, the thing that enables you to be faster at your projects when you're not multitasking is the mindset, and we often don't realize how much mindset comes into play. When you are going back and forth from one project to another, you are in a different mental state going into another project which takes time to build and break. So, by the time you have managed to get into the mindset of project A you are already moving into project B, it is always

95

best that you devote your time and energy one project at a time if you want it to doe did an at a faster pace.

Set yourself a goal (time, quality, etc.)

All in all, multitasking will do you no good. It will only make you slower at your work and make you less productive. Making sure you stop multitasking is essential, as it will only help you live a better life. One thing to remember from this chapter is to put all your energy at one thing at a time, and this will yield you a lot of better projects or anything that you are working towards to be great. If you want to be more successful and live a better life, you need to make sure your projects are quality as I can't stress this point enough. You are probably reading this book because you want to get better at living your life or achieve goals that you just haven't yet, one of the reasons why you are not living the life that you want or haven't reached your goal could be a lot of things but, one of the items could be the quality of your work which could be taking a hit because of you multitasking. So, review yourself, and find out why you haven't achieved your goal and why you are not living the life that you want.

Then if you happen to stumble upon multitasking being the limiting factor or the quality of your work, I want you to stop multitasking and start working on one project at a time while giving it your full attention. What you will notice is that your work will have a higher quality and will be completed in a quicker amount of time following the steps listed above, which will change your life and help you achieve your life goals in a better more efficient way.

After reading this chapter, many might be thinking that this is more of a self-help book than it is a fasting book. The Truth is that we want you to understand how to live a better life by changing the habits that you are currently following. Truth be told, following intermittent fasting and making it a lifestyle is a lot more work than you think it is. For you to make it easy, you need to understand that you need to change your habits in order to be successful at fasting, which means you need to change the way you move the way you think and the way you perform. This chapter gives you a clear idea on how to start living a better life by changing up your habits, once you do change your practices you will notice that following the Intermittent fasting as a whole will be very easy for you. The reason why it will be straightforward for you is that you will change the way you move and the change the way you live your life in general. Changing the way you live your life will not only help you get better results, but it will also help you to follow fasting and to make it a lifestyle, many people confuse fasting as not being a part of a lifestyle, they don't realize that it needs to be a lifestyle for it to be a health benefit, and it is something that they're supporting to better their health. But the truth is that when they're following, you want to be healthier then you need to make sure that you're taking care of your health 24/7 365 days a year. Which means you need to make this a lifestyle, and for you to make this a lifestyle, we need to understand some self-help techniques to keep it sustained for a more extended period. Which is why this chapter is more self-help oriented, we wanted to make sure that this book is different from any other books that you've read when it comes to following the Intermittent fasting. The way we're going to be delivering it is by showing you how to change your lifestyle for the better instead of the worst. We're not just going to give you foods to eat and how to follow the Intermittent fasting, but in fact, we're going to change the way you eat overall and to make it a better experience for you once you start getting into fasting. With that being said, I hope this chapter was helpful to you, and we will see you in the next chapter.

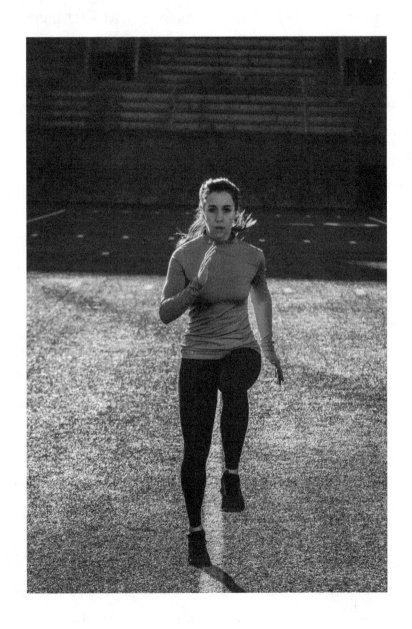

Chapter 7: Intermittent Fasting and Fitness

When following intermittent fasting, you have to keep in mind that even though you are eating very healthy and that you are taking care of your body having a good workout routine is recommended. Once you figured out what kind of intermittent fasting plan you're going to be following, make sure that you get a workout plan that will help you to put on muscle or lose body fat whichever your goal is.

One of the great amazing things about intermittent fasting is that you can lose weight or gain muscle while following this method, which is why many people consider intermittent fasting one of the best eating plans to follow, for overall health and wellness. By now, you know everything about intermittent fasting and how you should be following, especially for women as it is different from men when it comes to intermittent fasting. To understand how to stay healthy when intermittent fasting, there are some things you need to take care of before you start intermittent fasting. The first one would be to make sure that you have a proper workout plan based on your goals, there are many workout plans which you can find online that will help you to come up with a workout plan based on your goals. Keep in mind that you will have to work hard to come up with a workout plan if you're not an expert. If you can afford to get a personal trainer, then get one, as it will help you create a great workout plan for your needs. However, finding a workout plan online isn't so hard, and you can do so by looking up online for a bit.

Another aspect you need to make sure when intermittent fasting is that you need to take care of your diet, even though you are allowed to eat whatever you want when intermittent fasting you need to make sure that your diet is a lot healthier if your goal is to lose weight. Don't get me wrong, and you will still lose weight when following intermittent fasting; however, making sure that you are eating very healthy, then you will see better results overall. Finally, you need to make sure that you're taking care of yourself internally. Make sure they are getting enough micronutrients throughout the day to support your health.

Another thing to keep in mind would be that you will lose fat most of the time when fasting instead of the weight. Keep in mind, and When fasting, you will gain muscle and lose fat, which might not make you lose weight but instead fat. As always do body measurements instead of bodyweight check overall.

There are many ways to go about it, but one of the best ways to go about it would be to take multivitamins during your eating window. Keep in mind that if you take multivitamins when you are fasting will break the fast, so make sure that you're not taking multivitamins during your fast but in fact after your fast. Finally, make sure that you do everything in conjunction if your goal is to see amazing results. There is no better way to see results, and if you combine all three aspects, then you will be in a much better place to truly reap the benefits out of it.

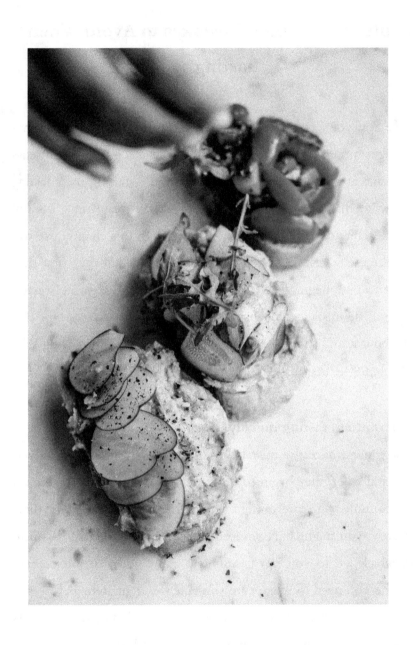

Chapter 8: Common Mistakes to Avoid When Fasting

We now come to the final chapter of this book, and I hope it has been a remarkable journey for all of you as it is about to discuss the last topic at hand. Many people who are just starting their fasting cycle, tend to make beginners mistake, which can result in goals not being achieved and many other hosts of things. In this chapter, we will go over the main mistakes most beginners make when they first start fasting. If you are beginning with intermittent fasting, chances are you will make those mistakes. Meaning, for it to not happen, it is best that we talk about it and show you ways to combat it. With that being said, let's talk about the first mistake.

Start intermittent fasting quickly

Many beginners make the mistake of starting intermittent fasting way too fast, and when they begin to quickly, it becomes unsustainable for them to continue with intermittent fasting. If you have started anything immediately, you might have noticed that it became tough for you to follow, which led to you not continuing. Same goes for intermittent fasting, and you need to make sure you take the right steps before you jump into following intermittent fasting. With that being said, let's talk about many ways beginner intermittent fasters tend to start too quickly.

The first mistake they make is by picking a fasting protocol, which is way out of their Realm.

As we talked about before, you need to ease into intermittent fasting, especially if you're women. You cannot expect to fast for 24 hours when you have never even fasted in your life, so start small. It is always recommended that women begin with 12-hour fast, or if that sounds too intense for you can start to by meal skipping. You have to make sure that, whatever you follow it is done gradually, so you don't quit. Another way people tend to start intermittent fasting too quickly is by not Consulting the doctor. Believe it or not, their chances that you might not be healthy enough to follow intermittent fasting.

That is why it is advised that you consult a doctor before starting fasting; for example, if you have diabetes, you are not advised to begin intermittent fasting. There are many health complications which not allow you to follow intermittent fasting, that is why we always recommend you ask a doctor before you start intermittent fasting or it can be very devastating.

Beginners also tend to extend the fasting window very quickly; if you haven't fasted for more than four weeks comfortably, then it is not recommended to extend the fasting window. We need to take into consideration that for beginners, going from 12 hours to 16 hours can be a drastic difference. That is why it is always advised that you stick with a fasting protocol for an extended period, ideally for four weeks. If you make the jump of increasing hours too soon, you will notice it becomes tough for you to continue with fasting and you might give up.

Choose the wrong plan for your lifestyle

Most people, when they first start intermittent fasting, tend to pick the crazy strategy for their lifestyle. It is important that you choose the right method for your lifestyle and your goals. Intermittent fasting can be very fitting for most lifestyle. However, some plans are just better suited for some. Which is what we are going to be talking about in this section of the book, picking the right plan for your lifestyle. To simplify this process, we will make up two people and make up a fake lifestyle.

Once we have managed to do that, we will figure out which fasting protocol works best for them. The first example would be Jamie, and she is the CEO of a company. Her daily routine is, she wakes up at 5 am and heads on out to her office. She works for 10 hours a day, in and out of meetings and has barely enough time to go to the bathroom. Her job is physically demanding, and it is also very mentally demanding.

Her goal is to lose a little weight, and she also wants more mental clarity since she has been noticing mental fog sometimes. According to Jamie's lifestyle, it is highly recommended that she follows a fasting protocol which requires less than 24 hours of fasting and is supported regularly. The reason behind her fasting less than 24 hours, is that when you fast for longer than 24 hours, you tend to notice diminishing results in energy. Which is not something we want for Jamie since she has to run a company. On the other hand, she wants less mental fog and more focus.

As you know, fasting for 12 to 20 hours has shown to increase mental focus, which would make a protocol 16/8 or the 12 hours fast more feasible for Jamie. She also wanted to lose weight, which can be done following the 16 hours quickly. In future, if Jamie wants to lose more weight without losing mental focus, then she can do that by following the warrior diet instead merely because it will shorten her eating window putting here in a higher caloric deficit. To summarize, Jamie's goal was to gain more mental clarity and energy while losing some fat. Her lifestyle is very demanding.

Hence, she is required to be on her "A game" every day, which is why the 12-hour fast or the 16-hour fast will work tremendously, as it has shown to help with mental energy and losing weight. If your lifestyle sounds similar to Jamie's, then I would highly recommend you follow the 12 hours fast or the 16 hours fast. For the next case study, we will pick Amanda. She has two kids, and she works part-time. Her main goal is to lose weight as quickly as possible, but healthily, she has gained a lot of weight after her last pregnancy. Her daily lifestyle is very sedentary since her kids are not infants anymore; taking care of them is more comfortable.

She works from home part-time, and her job is straightforward going. She has had experience with fasting before, she has followed the 12 hours fast and the 16 hours fasts both for four weeks. But now she is dangerous, and she wants to lose a ton of weight quickly. Since Amanda has experience with intermittent fasting, she can go right ahead and follow the two days a week fasting protocol or the alternate day fasting protocol; these two will put her in a 20%-25% deficit for the whole week making her lose weight quickly and in a healthy manner.

To sum up, Amanda, she has a very sedentary lifestyle. Her goal is to lose the pregnancy weight quickly and to do it healthily, she has followed the 12 hours fast and the 16 hours fast before. Based on her goals and lifestyle ideally, she can start with the alternate fasting protocol or the two days a week fasting protocol. If your goals and lifestyle sound very similar to Amanda's, then you should follow the two days a week fasting protocol or the alternate day fasting protocol. Hopefully, these two examples helped you understand which fasting protocol is best suited for your lifestyle. Just remember that fasting will only help you if you can do it for a sustained period, which is why lifestyle plays a huge role in sustainability for intermittent fasting. Pick your fasting protocols accordingly

Overeat during the eating window or too little

People make the mistake of eating a lot or too little when following intermittent fasting, and the truth is it is straightforward to do either. People who are looking to lose weight will eat less during their eating window, thinking that it will help you lose more body fat. Whereas overeating will not make up for all the fasting, you did throughout the day. Which is why it is imperative that you do none, so in this section, we will teach you how to make sure you aren't doing either when following an intermittent fasting protocol.

The first way to not mess up on overeating would be to make sure that you are counting your macros. This is one of the best ways to make sure you stay on track with your eating habits during your fasting windows. When you have calculated your macros and following them accordingly, you will have a lot better chance of not under eating or overeating during your eating window. Another way to make sure that you are not overeating is to eat slowly, and many people tend to get extremely excited when they see food in front of them during their eating window. It is best advised that you don't indulge in them and more than you should.

That is why it is essential that you control your cravings; we have taught you how to do that in the previous chapters. Now, even though fasting allows you to eat whatever you want when you break your fast, it still essential to make sure you eat correctly. You see if you try and eat junk food and try and hit your macros, it would be tough for you not to overeat. Let me explain how that works, as there is something called a high glycemic carb which most of the junk foods. What these high glycemic carbs are responsible for is digesting very quickly in your body, which spikes the insulin very fast.

When you absorb and shuttle the foods to quickly as you would with junk food, you will get hungry very fast, which would make you overeat. Which is why it is best advised that you eat foods which have a lower glycemic index like most healthy meals tend to have. Another thing these healthy foods will help you with would be the fiber, making you feel fuller through the day. Now that we know how not to overeat, let's talk about how to make sure that you aren't under-eating. The first way to make sure that you aren't under-eating would be by counting macros, and this will help you make sure that you are hitting all your calories for the day. Counting macros will ensure you don't under-eat and you don't overeat, it goes hand in hand.

Now, this is the only way to avoid under-eating let's talk about some of the signs you might be experiencing if you under-eat when fasting. The first sign you might notice is that you feel very weak when working out if you follow a workout plan you will see that your strength has gone down which is a tail-tail sign that you are under-eating. Another way to tell that you are under-eating is if you know that you feel less energy throughout the day, rather than feeling more heat. One of the many benefits of intermittent fasting is the fact that you can get a lot more power, but it won't work if you are under-eating. So by now, you can tell that overeating and under-eating aren't optimal for fasting. Which is why you need to make sure that you stay on track with your macros when fasting, the other tips we gave you work great as well.

But do whatever works for you to ensure that you aren't under eating or overeating, and there are millions of way to go about it. Find an eating routine which helps you feel full, and allows you to eat just the right amount of calories to where you are getting closer to your goals instead of drifting away from them if your goal is weight loss or muscle gains you need to make sure your calories are the right amount. Don't make this beginners mistake as you will regret it, and now you have the tools to ensure you don't make these mistakes.

Ignore what for when

One mistake that many people following intermittent fasting make is to ignore what for when. For you to be successful with intermittent fasting, you need to make sure you don't overlook what for when. What do I mean by what for when is simple, ignoring what to do and what not to do when intermittent fasting. We will talk about things to avoid and the things not to avoid when intermittent fasting. More specifically, we will teach you how to listen to your body.

You are ignoring what for when is merely a metaphor, nonetheless an important one. First of all, when intermittent fasting doesn't jump too quickly from fasts to fasts. Most beginners make the mistake of not riding out the protocol for a substantial amount of time before they jump to conclusions. Make sure that you have done at least four weeks of

111

following this protocol as it will show you how your body reacts to this fasting method. The next thing to make sure of would be to understand how your body reacts to certain types of fasting, as it is essential that you know so.

Before you jump the guns of upping the fasting difficultly, make sure you know how your body works. You need to remember that your body is more important than your goals, so whatever you do, you need to be aware of what your body is telling you. Don't do anything which makes you feel like you are harming your body, and as always consult with your physician before you start a fast.

Not drinking enough water

Drinking water is crucial when your intermittent fasting, is there a lot of benefits to drinking water. It also helps you care about your appetite. We will talk about the reasons why you should be drinking more water when intermittent fasting, and also show you why you might not be drinking enough water and techniques to allow you to drink more water when fasting. Many people know that water is very beneficial to humans, water help to detox your body clean out your system and also helps you curb appetite. It is crucial that you're drinking more water when fasting. Believe it or not, most of the time you're drinking a lot less water than you required to be drinking. One of the best rules of thumb to follow when you are drinking water is too drink 1 oz per pound of body weight. So if you weigh 150 lbs., you should be drinking 150 ounces of water, especially when you're intermittent fasting; as water will help you forget about food.

Many people know that when you're fasting, especially in the beginning you tend to crave a lot of food. What water will do is help you curb that appetite, so you don't break you're fast prematurely, another thing water will do detoxify your body. When your fasting you're already detoxing a lot of things, if you add more water to it, it will help you detox your body even further making it a lot healthier environment for you. Water will also increase your brain power and productivity, as you know intermittent fasting has shown to improve mental focus so once you add more water to your daily routine, you will notice more focused throughout the day.

Another thing water helps you with is that it helps you lose body weight. If you started intermittent fasting in the hopes of losing weight, then you need to drink more water. What water does, is it increase your metabolism, which equals more calories burnt throughout the day. Water will also help you clean out your complexion, so if that's what you're looking for the water will help you with that. Intermittent fasting has shown to improve with your digestive system, but once you add a sufficient amount of water to it will boost it further. Many people know that regularity in the essential thing when it comes to a healthy body, why do I help you with consistency, which will equal a better digestive system and overall well-being. Water will also help you boost your immune system, as it enables you to clean out your toxins.

When incorporated with intermittent fasting, drink more water to boost your immune system. When fasting, you might notice headaches, especially in the beginning, if you drink a sufficient amount of water throughout the day, you will not see problems. Headaches is one of the biggest concerns when fasting, many people notice problems, and to avoid that you should start drinking more water. Another matter that you might see when fasting is cramped more specifically muscle cramps. One of the ways to prevent it is to drink more water. Now I can keep going on with the benefits of drinking more water, but you get the idea to drink more water to avoid side effects from fasting that you might see. One of the ways to ensure that you drink more water is to buy a water bottle with markings on it. First, figure out how much water you need through the day and make sure you achieve your goal of drinking a set amount of water. Another way to ensure that you drink more water is to set alarms. What many people do, set alerts on this Smartphone, and when the alarm goes off the drink a glass of water. You can do the same thing to ensure they drink enough water throughout the day, calculate the number of glasses you need to achieve your water intake goal, and then set your timer.

Choose whichever method you want to make sure that you're drinking enough water throughout the day. Not drinking enough water is one of the biggest mistakes most people make. Our body is made up of around 70% water, and to ignore that and not drink enough water and hinder your progress. Make sure you're drinking enough water, during your fast and after you break your fast. To ensure that you are optimizing your fasting endeavors and getting closer to your goals.

We have now officially completed the book. I hope you learned a lot from it as it was our goal to ensure that no stones where unturned. This final chapter has to be one of the most important ones, as it helps you figure out any mistakes you might make in the beginning. Many books don't cover mistakes which beginners might make when following intermittent fasting, and that is why we had to write a chapter, especially on it.

We understand that fasting can be confusing and hard at first, so it is essential that you are aware of the mistakes you might or might not make. Please make sure that you have understood all the things you should so and the things you shouldn't be doing. Just be aware of the fact that there might be many things which might go wrong in the beginning, learn from your mistakes, and keep moving on forward.

Don't let small mistakes stop you from achieving your dream body, and helping you live a healthier life overall. If you need extra motivation, ask a friend to keep you on track, always let them know how important it is for you to not give up on this journey. But once again, listen to your body if you feel like fasting is harming your body then stop as your body is more important than anything else, which is why we recommend getting blood work done by a professional always before you start any plan. As always, thanks for reading this book.

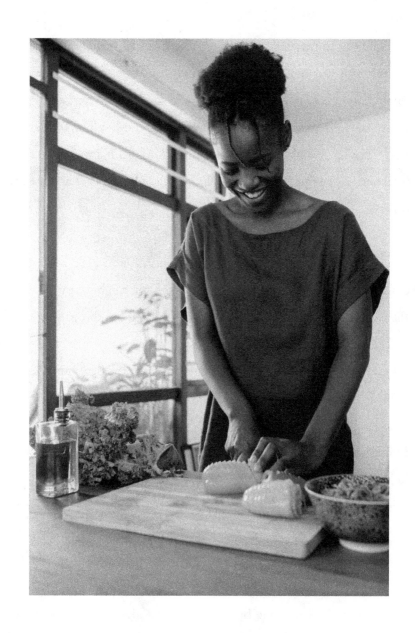

Conclusion

Thank you so much for downloading the book *Intermittent Fasting for Women*. As you can tell, we learned a lot in this book, not only did we talk about intermittent fasting and how it affects women but we also talked about how to follow intermittent fasting the right way when you are a woman. Keep in mind that being a woman and following intermittent fasting is a lot different from men, as you can tell by reading this book.

Not only that, but we also helped you to figure out which intermittent fasting protocol will be the right one to follow based on your goals and how to get the most out of it. Overall, this book was a complete package when it comes to delivering the right information to women in terms of following intermittent fasting. Keep in mind that if you understand all the information provided to you in this book, you will be in a much better place to follow intermittent fasting and to see the benefits from it.

Overall, make sure that you consult with your doctor before you follow any intermittent fasting protocols as it can be different effects for you. With that being said, hopefully, you enjoyed the information provided to you in this book, and we hope that you learned a lot from it. With that being said, leave is an excellent review if you enjoyed the information provided to you and as always learn from this book and apply the knowledge as soon as possible.